Evidence-Based Laryngology

David E. Rosow • Chandra M. Ivey
Editors

Evidence-Based Laryngology

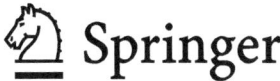 Springer

Editors
David E. Rosow
Department of Otolaryngology
University of Miami Miller
School of Medicine
Miami, FL
USA

Chandra M. Ivey
Department of Otolaryngology
Head and Neck Surgery
Icahn School of Medicine at
Mount Sinai
New York, NY
USA

ISBN 978-3-030-58493-1   ISBN 978-3-030-58494-8   (eBook)
https://doi.org/10.1007/978-3-030-58494-8

This Springer imprint is published by the registered company Springer Nature Switzerland AG
The registered company address is: Gewerbestrasse 11, 6330 Cham, Switzerland

I dedicate this work to the memory of my father, Carl Rosow, MD, PhD, the greatest role model I could ask for, whose professional mantra was always "show me the evidence."

—David E. Rosow, MD, FACS

I would like to acknowledge my children, Maddock and Caitlin Marsallo, who fuel my gratitude and inspire my curiosity and passion daily.

—Chandra M. Ivey, MD, FACS

Preface

How do we make clinical decisions in laryngology? It may seem like an overly broad question, but the answer usually boils down to one of four options:

1. My fellowship director told me.
2. I read a paper on it once.
3. In my experience, this works best for me.
4. I personally conducted a systematic review of all available high-quality literature on this topic, synthesizing multiple randomized, double-blinded, placebo-controlled trials to arrive at my conclusion.

This is an obvious oversimplification, but it does emphasize how frequently the answer is one of the first three options and how rarely we can choose Option 4. Despite the long history of our field, we have been slow to adopt the tenets of practicing evidence-based medicine, with many of our decisions guided by retrospective case series and expert opinions.

Evidence-based medicine is defined as the application of the best-available (i.e., most reliable) evidence gained from the scientific method to guide clinical decision-making [1]. One early description of evidence-based medicine noted that our recommended treatment policies must be tied to "evidence instead of standard-of-care practices or the beliefs of experts." [2]

There are many ratings scales that can be used to determine the quality of evidence in a published research paper. The Oxford University Centre for Evidence-Based Medicine maintains probably the best-known rating system, and for this text, we will use a simplified version of this system [3].

Level 1	Randomized controlled trials (RCTs) Meta-analysis or systematic review of RCTs showing consistent results
Level 2	Prospective comparative studies Meta-analysis or systematic review of Level 1 or 2 studies with inconsistent results
Level 3	Retrospective cohort studies Case control studies Meta-analysis or systematic review of Level 3 studies
Level 4	Case series Cross-sectional survey study
Level 5	Case report, expert opinion, personal observation

Please note that this system does not automatically mean that higher level evidence is necessarily "better"; there are many factors that go into determining the quality of research, and this is only a simple guide. For example, an observational study with a large number of subjects and significant treatment effect is potentially more useful than a Cochrane review of a few small studies with no conclusive result. Furthermore, there are areas of medicine that are not amenable to randomized control trials. One frequently told joke holds that there are no placebo-controlled trials of the effects of using a parachute when jumping out of an airplane, so how can we *really* know that they work?

Keeping all this in mind, we have sought to create a manual for otolaryngologists, residents, speech-language pathologists, and any other clinicians who manage laryngological problems and would like to know the evidence basis behind different treatment options. This is purposefully not a comprehensive reference textbook—there are many well-written ones currently available—but to the best of our knowledge, they do not focus specifically on the evidence justification for their statements.

Each chapter in a reference text may have dozens of references, which can make casual browsing through the evidence difficult. In this book, we have sought to summarize the key evidence for each section in boxes such as the following:

Level of evidence	Conclusion
2	Prospective cohort data shows muscle tension dysphonia (MTD) may be a marker of vocal fold paralysis/paresis

We recognize that the value of research cannot be easily distilled into a single number, but recommend readers use this text simply as a guide concerning current laryngology practices. We expect practitioners to decide for themselves if there is a significant evidence basis to support their personal clinical decisions; this book strives to make it more efficient and convenient to do so.

Miami, FL, USA   David E. Rosow, MD
New York, NY, USA   Chandra M. Ivey, MD

References

1. Evidence based medicine. (n.d.) Segen's Medical Dictionary. (2011). Retrieved 29 June 2020.
2. Eddy DM. Practice policies: guidelines for methods. JAMA. 1990;263(13):1839–41.
3. OCEBM Levels of Evidence Working Group. The Oxford 2011 levels of evidence. Oxford Centre for Evidence-Based Medicine. http://www. cebm.net/index.aspx?o=5653. Retrieved 29 June 2020.

Contents

Contributors

James W. Bao, BA Department of Otolaryngology, University of Miami Miller School of Medicine, Miami, FL, USA

Andrew Blitzer, MD, DDS Department of Otolaryngology, Head and Neck Surgery, Columbia University College of Physicians and Surgeons, New York, NY, USA

Keith A. Chadwick, MD The Sean Parker Institute for the Voice, Department of Otolaryngology-Head & Neck Surgery, Weill Cornell Medical College – New York Presbyterian Hospital, New York, NY, USA

Christopher D. Dwyer, MD UCSF Voice and Swallowing Center, Department of Otolaryngology-Head and Neck Surgery, University of California, San Francisco, San Francisco, CA, USA

Chandra M. Ivey, MD Department of Otolaryngology, Head and Neck Surgery, Icahn School of Medicine at Mount Sinai, New York, NY, USA

Gauri Kapre, MBBS, MS (ENT) Neeti Clinics Pvt Ltd, Department of ENT, Nagpur, Maharashtra, India

Diana N. Kirke, MD Department of Otolaryngology, Head and Neck Surgery, Icahn School of Medicine at Mount Sinai, New York, NY, USA

Juliana K. Litts, MA, CCC-SLP Department of Otolaryngology, University of Colorado School of Medicine, Aurora, CO, USA

Patrick O. McGarey Jr, MD Department of Otolaryngology, Head and Neck Surgery, University of Virginia Health System, Charlottesville, VA, USA

Nupur Kapoor Nerurkar, MBBS, MS (ENT) Head- Bombay Hospital Voice and Swallowing Center, Bombay Hospital, Mumbai, India

Ashli O'Rourke, MS, MD Evelyn Trammell Institute for Voice & Swallowing, Department of Otolaryngology - Head and Neck Surgery, Medical University of South Carolina, Charleston, SC, USA

Debbie R. Pan, MD Department of Head and Neck Surgery & Communication Sciences, Duke University, Durham, NC, USA

David E. Rosow, MD Department of Otolaryngology, University of Miami Miller School of Medicine, Miami, FL, USA

Angelina Schache, MS, CCC-SLP Department of Otolaryngology - Head and Neck Surgery, University of Washington School of Medicine, Seattle, WA, USA

C. Blake Simpson, MD UAB Voice Center, Department of Otolaryngology, University of Alabama-Birmingham, Birmingham, AL, USA

Lucian Sulica, MD The Sean Parker Institute for the Voice, Department of Otolaryngology-Head & Neck Surgery, Weill Cornell Medical College – New York Presbyterian Hospital, New York, NY, USA

Abhishek Vaidya, MBBS, MS (ENT) National Cancer Institute, Department of Head and Neck Surgery, Nagpur, Maharashtra, India

VyVy N. Young, MD UCSF Voice and Swallowing Center, Department of Otolaryngology-Head and Neck Surgery, University of California, San Francisco, San Francisco, CA, USA

Fermin M. Zubiaur, MD Otorhinolaryngology Surgical Group, Panamericana University School of Medicine, Mexico City, Mexico

Vocal Fold Nodules

1

Patrick O. Mcgarey Jr
and C. Blake Simpson

Introduction

While there is no universally accepted nomenclature system for benign vocal fold lesions, vocal fold nodules (VFNs) are defined as bilateral, mid-membranous vocal fold lesions that respond to voice therapy (Fig. 1.1) [1]. They are the most common organic laryngeal pathology seen in professional voice users and voice patients overall, identified in 15% of patients presenting with dysphonia [2]. A national South Korean health survey reported a 1.3% prevalence of VFN in men and women >19 years old [3].

VFNs are characterized histopathologically by epithelial hyperplasia, basement membrane thickening, and fibrosis. These lesions are contained within the basement membrane zone and superficial lamina propria [4]. VFNs contain dense organizations of fibronectin [5], a molecule that plays an important role in

P. O. Mcgarey Jr (✉)
Department of Otolaryngology, Head and Neck Surgery,
University of Virginia Health System, Charlottesville, VA, USA
e-mail: pmcgarey@virginia.edu; POM4FB@hscmail.mcc.virginia.edu

C. B. Simpson
UAB Voice Center, Department of Otolaryngology,
University of Alabama-Birmingham, Birmingham, AL, USA

© Springer Nature Switzerland AG 2021   1
D. E. Rosow, C. M. Ivey (eds.), *Evidence-Based Laryngology*,
https://doi.org/10.1007/978-3-030-58494-8_1

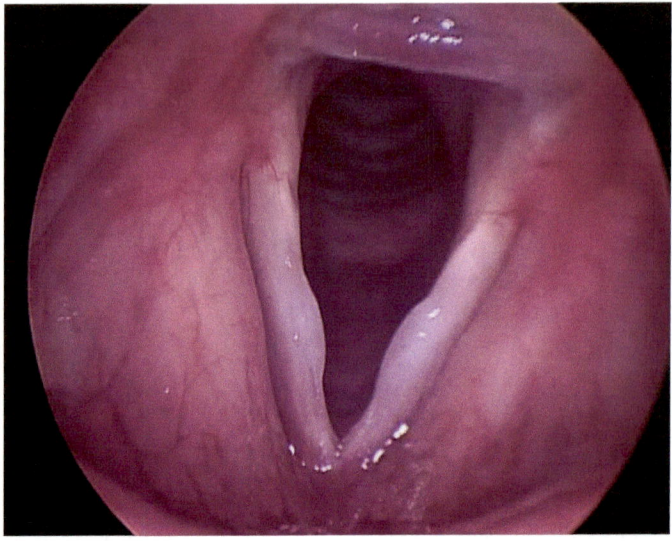

Fig. 1.1 Vocal fold nodules viewed by laryngeal videostroboscopy

wound healing and tissue remodeling [6], and is thought to be a precursor for collagen formation [7].

Etiology and Diagnosis

VFNs develop in the setting of phonotrauma. Jiang and Titze demonstrated that the mid-membranous portion of the vocal fold receives the maximum impact stress during phonation, helping to establish the relationship between most mid-membranous lesions and phonotrauma [8]. In one study of 221 patients with benign vocal fold lesions, 80% occurred at the mid-membranous location [9]. Not surprisingly, occupation is a risk factor for development of voice disorders, including VFNs. Heavy vocal use professions are at highest risk, including not only singers, actors, and other performing artists, but also teachers and other educators, social workers, counselors, clergy, and lawyers [10, 11]. The majority of VFNs occur in young females. Zhukhovitskaya et al. revealed that roughly 90% of VFNs identified in a voice clinic were in female patients, and roughly 85% in patients 18–39 years of age [12]. Extroverted personality has been associated with VFNs [13]. Bouchayer et al. reported on over 500 patients with nodules who underwent surgery and found a small congenital anterior glottic web in 22% of cases, the significance of which is unknown [14]. While laryngopharyngeal reflux (LPR) has been shown to occur more often in patients with VFNs compared to controls [15], pepsin is generally not present in VFNs excision specimens [16]. It is conceivable that in some patients, the chronic cough and throat clearing associated with gastroesophageal reflux disease (GERD) and LPR could contribute to vocal fold trauma leading to development of VFNs, although this is more commonly associated with posterior laryngeal pathology such as granuloma [17].

Vocal fold nodules are typically identified on laryngeal videostroboscopy as bilateral lesions, which are most often symmetric. VFNs have normal or minimally impaired mucosal wave. They are also defined by their response to non-operative treatment, specifically vocal hygiene, management of comorbid conditions contributing to laryngeal inflammation, and voice therapy [1].

Level of evidence	Conclusion
4	Retrospective studies show that VFNs occur primarily at the mid-membranous vocal fold and are more common in children and young adults, vocal professionals, females, and extroverted personality types [9, 10, 12, 13]

Treatment

Conservative Treatment

Behavioral therapy including behavioral education, laryngeal hygiene, and voice therapy has been shown to be effective in improving vocal function in patients with VFNs, with treatment success rates ranging from 88% to 100% [18–21]. It is important to note that the definition of treatment success varies greatly, and many studies did not assess patients with laryngeal videostroboscopy after treatment. It has been shown that while vocal function and voice quality often improve with behavioral treatment and voice therapy, complete regression of vocal fold lesions after treatment was low in several reports [22–25]. In addition, one study found no difference in short- and long-term VHI-10, perceptual voice evaluation scores, and acoustic parameters between patients with remnant nodules and those with a complete lesion response after treatment with voice therapy [25]. A meta-analysis of studies assessing acoustic voice parameters before and after voice therapy for treatment of VFNs showed a statistically significant improvement in fundamental frequency and jitter after treatment [26].

Level of evidence	Conclusion
3	Voice therapy is an effective intervention for improving voice quality in the setting of VFNs, despite the fact that oftentimes the lesions do not fully resolve [19–21]

Given the lack of availability of voice therapists in some medical settings, a Japanese study sought to evaluate the effectiveness of a vocal hygiene education program consisting of an individualized private short lecture (by a physician or voice therapist) followed by standardized videotaped lessons. This study randomized participants with VFNs and vocal fold polyps (VFPs) to receive this education program or the standard basic laryngeal hygiene education. Although the results reported VFNs and VFPs together, there was a combined 61.3% lesion resolution rate in the treatment group compared to 26.3% ($p < 0.001$) in the standard education group. In addition, the rate of lesion resolution for VFNs was higher (OR 4.8, $P < 0.001$) compared to VFP, although the individual data was not reported for each lesion type [27].

Level of evidence	Conclusion
1	Intensive laryngeal hygiene education can be effective in lesion resolution in patient with VFNs and decreases the need for surgery [27]

Voice therapy via telepractice is gaining popularity, especially in the wake of the COVID-19 pandemic, and there is evidence for its use in VFNs and other voice disorders. A randomized trial demonstrated similar efficacy of voice therapy via telepractice compared to in-person voice therapy in the treatment of muscle tension dysphonia [28]. Fu et al. demonstrated the efficacy of this practice in the treatment of 10 women with VFNs using video conferencing technology. After an initial vocal hygiene education session face-to-face in the clinic, patients underwent eight sessions of voice therapy via telepractice. Perceptual, stroboscopic, acoustic, and physiologic assessments were made by a blinded speech language pathologist and an otolaryngologist. Results were similar when compared to results from a separate group of patients treated with conventional face-to-face intensive voice therapy by the same group of clinicians [29].

Level of evidence	Conclusion
3	Voice therapy via telepractice has comparable efficacy to conventional in-office voice therapy in the treatment of VFNs [29]

Surgical Treatment

While non-surgical interventions are the mainstay of treatment of VFNs, surgical therapy can be entertained in selected patients who fail initial therapy. A Cochrane review first performed in

2001 and last updated in 2012 sought to compare the effectiveness of surgical vs. non-surgical therapy for VFNs. No suitable trials were identified [30]. Béquignon et al. (2013) retrospectively analyzed a group of 62 patients who had undergone surgical therapy for VFNs, with or without postoperative voice therapy. The rate of recurrent dysphonia without postoperative voice therapy was 56%, compared to 22% for those receiving postoperative voice therapy. Recurrent dysphonia, when it occurred, was noted at a mean interval of 5.2 years after surgery, and new vocal fold pathology (VFNs or polypoid corditis) was seen in 18% of patients [31]. This study highlights that while surgery can remove VFNs successfully, addressing the underlying behavioral etiology of this condition is critical to treatment success.

Level of evidence	Conclusion
4	In those patient requiring surgery for VFNs, postoperative voice therapy reduces recurrence of dysphonia and phonotraumatic vocal fold lesions [31]

There are other non-surgical modalities for the treatment of VFNs. Woo et al. demonstrated a 42% complete resolution rate among 33 patients with VFNs who underwent percutaneous subepithelial steroid injection after refusing voice therapy and surgery. Their recurrence rate was low (3%), but long-term follow-up was lacking [32]. Wang et al. performed a retrospective review of adults with VFNs and vocal fold polyp (VFP), comparing vocal hygiene education to in-office vocal fold steroid injection. Comparing 33 patients with VFNs treated with vocal fold steroid injection, lesion size improved to a greater extent with steroid injection at 1 month, but both steroid injection and vocal hygiene groups had comparable lesion size reduction at 2 months (37% reduction for steroid group, 26% reduction for vocal hygiene group) [33]. Long-term follow-up of 72 patients with VFNs treated by this same laryngology group with in-office vocal fold steroid injection demonstrated only a 31% failure rate (symptom recurrence or need for additional intervention) at 2 years [34]. Additional research is needed to characterize the role of steroid injection in the management of VFNs.

Level of evidence	Conclusion
4	Office-based subepithelial injection of steroid can be an effective treatment for VFNs [32, 33]

Transcutaneous electrical nerve stimulation (TENS) is a well-established technique in the physical therapy field, and it has been studied as an adjunct to voice therapy for the treatment of voice disorders. Although there remains some controversy regarding its effectiveness [35], studies have demonstrated beneficial effects on pain pathways [36], local blood flow [37], and muscle relaxation [38]. Several studies combining this technique with standard voice therapy maneuvers have shown promising effects on glottic function in patients with VFNs [39, 40].

References

1. Rosen CA, Gartner-Schmidt J, Hathaway B, et al. A nomenclature paradigm for benign midmembranous vocal fold lesions. Laryngoscope. 2012;122(6):1335–41.
2. Van Houtte E, Van Lierde K, D'Haeseleer E, Claeys S. The prevalence of laryngeal pathology in a treatment-seeking population with dysphonia. Laryngoscope. 2010;120(2):306–12.
3. Woo SH, Kim RB, Choi SH, Lee SW, Won SJ. Prevalence of laryngeal disease in South Korea: data from the Korea national health and nutrition examination survey from 2008 to 2011. Yonsei Med J. 2014;55(2):499–507.
4. Martins RHG, Defaveri J, Domingues MAC, et al. Vocal fold nodules: morphological and immunohistochemical investigations. J Voice. 2010;24:531–9.
5. Courey MS, Shohet JA, Scott MA, Ossoff RH. Immunohistochemical characterization of benign laryngeal lesions. Ann Otol Rhinol Laryngol. 1996;105(7):525–31.

6. Grinnell F. Fibronectin and wound healing. J Cell Biochem. 1984;26(2):107–16.

7. Gray SD, Hammond E, Hanson DF. Benign pathologic responses of the larynx. Ann Otol Rhinol Laryngol. 1995;104:13–8.

8. Jiang JJ, Titze IR. Measurement of vocal fold intraglottal pressure and impact stress. J Voice. 1994;8(2):132–44.

9. Poels PJ, de Jong FI, Schutte HK. Consistency of the preoperative and intraoperative diagnosis of benign vocal fold lesions. J Voice. 2003;17(3):425–33.

10. Mori MC, Francis DO, Song PC. Identifying occupations at risk for laryngeal disorders requiring specialty voice care. Otolaryngol Head Neck Surg. 2017;157(4):670–5.

11. Fritzell B. Voice disorders and occupation. Logoped Phoniatr Vocol. 2009;21(1):7–12.

12. Zhukhovitskaya A, Battaglia D, Khosla SM, Murry T, Sulica L. Gender and age in benign vocal fold lesions. Laryngoscope. 2015;125(1):191–6.

13. Yano J, Ichimura K, Hoshino T, Nozue M. Personality factors in pathogenesis of polyps and nodules of vocal cords. Auris Nasus Larynx. 1982;9(2):105–10.

14. Bouchayer M, Cornut G. Microsurgical treatment of benign vocal fold lesions: indications, technique, results. Folia Phoniatr (Basel). 1992;44(3–4):155–84.

15. Kuhn J, Toohill RJ, Ulualp SO, et al. Pharyngeal acid reflux events in patients with vocal cord nodules. Laryngoscope. 1998;108(8 Pt 1):1146–9.

16. Tasli H, Eser B, Asik MB, Birkent H. Does pepsin play a role in etiology of laryngeal nodules? J Voice. 2019;33:704–7.

17. Ylitalo R, Ramel S. Extraesophageal reflux in patients with contact granuloma: a prospective controlled study. Ann Otol Rhinol Laryngol. 2002;111:441–6.

18. McFarlane SC, Watterson TL. Vocal nodules: endoscopic study of their variations and treatment. Semin Speech Lang. 1990;11:47–59.

19. Salturk Z, Ozdemir E, Sari H, et al. Assessment of resonant voice therapy in the treatment of vocal fold nodules. J Voice. 2019;33:810.e1–4.

20. Murry T, Woodson GE. A comparison of three methods for the management of vocal fold nodules. J Voice. 1992;6(3):271–6.

21. Mansuri B, Tohidast SA, Soltaninejad N, Kamali M, Ghelichi L, Azimi H. Nonmedical treatments of vocal fold nodules: a systematic review. J Voice. 2018;32(5):609–20.

22. Holmberg EB, Hillman RE, Hammarberg B, Södersten M, Doyle P. Efficacy of a behaviorally based voice therapy protocol for vocal nodules. Voice. 2001;15(3):395–412.

23. Chernobelsky SI. The treatment and results of voice therapy amongst professional classical singers with vocal fold nodules. Logoped Phoniatr Vocol. 2007;32(4):178–84.

24. Fu S, Theodoros DG, Ward EC. Intensive versus traditional voice therapy for vocal nodules: perceptual, physiological, acoustic and aerodynamic changes. J Voice. 2015;29(2):260, 31–44.

25. Jo YS, Kim MY, So YK. Impact of remnant nodules on immediate and long-term outcomes of voice therapy for vocal fold nodules. J Voice. 2019;S0892-1997:30316–9. Web. 18 June. 2020.
26. Alegria R, Freitas SV, Manso MC. Is there an improvement on acoustic voice parameters in patients with bilateral vocal fold nodules after voice therapy? A meta-analysis. Eur Arch Otorhinolaryngol. 2020;277:2163–72. Web. 18 June. 2020.
27. Hosoya M, Kobayashi R, Ishii T, et al. Vocal hygiene education program reduces surgical interventions for benign vocal fold lesions: a randomized controlled trial. Laryngoscope. 2018;128(11):2593–9.
28. Rangarathnam B, McCullough GH, Pickett H, Zraick RI, Tulunay-Ugur O, McCullough KC. Telepractice versus in-person delivery of voice therapy for primary muscle tension dysphonia. Am J Speech Lang Pathol. 2015;24(3):386–99.
29. Fu S, Theodoros DG, Ward EC. Delivery of intensive voice therapy for vocal fold nodules via telepractice: a pilot feasibility and efficacy study. J Voice. 2015;29(6):696–706.
30. Pedersen M, McGlashan J. Surgical versus non-surgical interventions for vocal cord nodules. Cochrane Database Syst Rev. 2001;(2).
31. Béquignon E, Bach C, Fugain C, et al. Long-term results of surgical treatment of vocal fold nodules. Laryngoscope. 2013;123(8):1926–30.
32. Woo JH, Kim DY, Kim JW, Oh EA, Lee SW. Efficacy of percutaneous vocal fold injections for benign laryngeal lesions: prospective multicenter study. Acta Otolaryngol. 2011;131(12):1326–32.
33. Wang CT, Liao LJ, Lai MS, Cheng PW. Comparison of benign lesion regression following vocal fold steroid injection and vocal hygiene education. Laryngoscope. 2014;124(2):510–5.
34. Wang CT, Lai MS, Cheng PW. Long-term surveillance following intralesional steroid injection for benign vocal fold lesions. JAMA Otolaryngol Head Neck Surg. 2017;143(6):589–94.
35. Sluka KA, Walsh DM. Transcutaneous electrical nerve stimulation: basic science mechanisms and clinical effectiveness. Pain. 2003;4:109–21.
36. Palmer S, Cramp F, Propert K, Godfrey H. Transcutaneous electrical nerve stimulation and transcutaneous spinal electroanalgesia: a preliminary efficacy and mechanisms-based investigation. Physiotherapy. 2009;95:185–91.
37. Sherry JE, Oehrlein KM, Hegge KS, Morgan BJ. Effect of burst-mode transcutaneous electrical nerve stimulation on peripheral vascular resistance. Phys Ther. 2001;81(6):1183–91.
38. Penkner K, Janda M, Lorenzoni MA. A comparison of the muscular relaxation effect of TENS and EMG-biofeedback in patients with bruxism. J Oral Rehabil. 2001;28:849–53.
39. Santos JK, Silvério KCA, Diniz Oliveira NFC, et al. Evaluation of electrostimulation effect in women with vocal nodules. J Voice. 2016;30:769.e1–7.
40. Silverio KCA, Brasolotto AG, Siqueira LTD, et al. Effect of application of transcutaneous electrical nerve stimulation and laryngeal manual therapy in dysphonic women: clinical trial. J Voice. 2015;29:200–8.

Recurrent Respiratory Papillomatosis

2

David E. Rosow and Chandra M. Ivey

Introduction

Recurrent respiratory papillomatosis (RRP) is an acquired condition resulting in the growth of exophytic, wart-like lesions anywhere in the upper aerodigestive tract. This chapter will solely focus on papillomatosis affecting the larynx, the most affected site. While RRP is a benign condition, its recurrent nature makes it a source of morbidity due to the frequent need for surgical debulking and rare potential for airway obstruction or malignant transformation. Management has evolved significantly over the last 50 years, and understanding the evidence basis for diagnostic and treatment approaches is critically important.

D. E. Rosow (✉)
Department of Otolaryngology, University of Miami Miller School of Medicine, Miami, FL, USA
e-mail: DRosow@med.miami.edu

C. M. Ivey
Department of Otolaryngology, Head and Neck Surgery, Icahn School of Medicine at Mount Sinai, New York, NY, USA

© Springer Nature Switzerland AG 2021
D. E. Rosow, C. M. Ivey (eds.), *Evidence-Based Laryngology*,
https://doi.org/10.1007/978-3-030-58494-8_2

Etiology and Pathogenesis

RRP is caused primarily by two strains of human papillomavirus (HPV), HPV-6 and HPV-11. HPV-11 is generally associated with more aggressive disease and higher potential for malignant transformation [1]. The disease has a bimodal distribution, with onset occurring both in children (approximately 4 per 100,000) and in adults (approximately 2 per 100,000) [2]. In spite of the relatively rare incidence, its recurrent nature leads to numerous surgical procedures, with an annual estimated cost to the US health care system of $200 million [3]. The average child requires nearly 20 procedures in their lifetime and an average of 4.4 per year, with over 15% of adults and children requiring over 40 lifetime procedures.

The exact mode of transmission is unknown. It is postulated that juvenile-onset RRP is transmitted vertically, from mother to child. Greater than 60% of women test positive for HPV antibodies, and anywhere from 1.5% to 5% of pregnant women in the USA are clinically infected, with a transmission risk in uncomplicated vaginal deliveries of approximately 1:400 for women with active cervical HPV [4]. Virus transmitted in this fashion may remain dormant and then activate during a period of immune decline or suppression.

Transmission may also occur horizontally, through sexual contact that may be orogenital or oral-anal in nature. Ruiz et al. [5] published a prospective case-control series demonstrating that greater than 25 lifetime sexual partners correlated with increased risk of developing RRP and that the median number of sexual partners was significantly higher in the RRP population than in controls (15 versus 10). In spite of this finding, it is very uncommon to find patients who infect their spouses or romantic partners, raising the question of whether host immunity or genetic factors play a role in viral expression [6].

Diagnosis

Visualization of the vocal folds and surrounding structures via laryngoscopy with or without stroboscopy is the primary method of diagnosis and surveillance in patients with RRP. There have been small studies demonstrating the feasibility of ultrasound in detecting papilloma in pediatric patients who may not tolerate endoscopy, but this is not a widely used technique [7]. Narrow-band imaging, which utilizes blue, filtered light to enhance detection of erythematous, vascular lesions, has been postulated to improve visualization of papilloma in areas that might be missed by white light [8]. It has been shown in one prospective study to increase the sensitivity of papilloma detection to 97%, up from 80% for plain, white light at the time of surgical microlaryngoscopy [9].

The Derkay score is the most widely used staging system for RRP, and it relies on rating laryngeal subsites as well as extralaryngeal areas for involvement with disease [10]. Though it was only validated with 17 pediatric patients in the original cohort, it was shown to predict surgical interval and has been subsequently been shown in a retrospective series to correlate with VHI-10 [11].

Level of evidence	Conclusion
3	Narrow-band imaging improves the sensitivity of papilloma detection compared to white light endoscopy [9]

Surgical Management

Traditional treatment of RRP has been surgical, and removal of most, if not all, diseased tissue has been a priority to prevent persistent infection and regrowth. This must be balanced at all times with the necessity of preserving laryngeal function, so avoidance of over-resection and unnecessary scarring are of paramount importance. The mainstays of surgical treatment of RRP for the last 50 years have been traditional microscopic instruments ("cold" technique) and surgical lasers. The CO_2 laser was introduced to laryngeal surgery in the early 1970s and had the advantage of reduced bleeding, though with the side effect of collateral thermal trauma to the microstructure of the vocal fold. Cold technique reduces this collateral damage at the expense of less hemostasis, but the introduction of powered microdebriders has enabled surgeons to "skim" papilloma from the epithelial surface while causing minimal disruption to the tissue underneath. A small, randomized prospective trial of 19 pediatric patients found no difference between CO_2 laser and microdebrider in postoperative pain, but found greater improvement in voice quality, shorter procedure times, and lower procedure cost [12].

Over time, the CO_2 laser has been gradually replaced with angiolytic lasers, first with the 585-nm pulsed-dye laser (PDL), then with the 532-nm potassium-titanyl-phosphate (KTP) laser [13, 14]. Both of these lasers work through the principle of selective photoangiolysis: their wavelengths correspond to absorption peaks for oxyhemoglobin, which allows vaporization of vascular targets while sparing surrounding tissue. Numerous studies have been published showing safety and efficacy in both OR and office environments, as well increased cost savings to health care systems when deployed in an office setting [14–16].

Adjuvant Treatment

Interferon-Alfa

The first widely used systemic treatment for RRP was interferon-alpha, which has been shown in some series to decrease the frequency of disease relapse in treated patients [17]. One randomized crossover trial of 66 pediatric patients was published twice separately in the same year after demonstrating some reduction in disease severity, though this effect was noted to diminish within 4 months of discontinuing treatment and was accompanied by elevation of liver function tests in 64% of patients [18, 19]. Healy et al. [20] performed a randomized control trial of 123 patients who received either surgery plus regular interferon treatments for 1 year or surgery alone. While there was significantly decreased growth rate of papilloma for the first 6 months, this effect disappeared afterward, and the authors concluded that interferon did not have significant benefit as a curative or adjuvant treatment.

Level of evidence	Conclusion
1	Randomized control trials show improved RRP severity initially with interferon alpha treatment, but this effect is short-lived [18]

Cidofovir

Cidofovir is an antiviral agent that is the most commonly used adjuvant treatment for RRP in children. It is FDA-approved only for IV therapy to prevent and treat cytomegalovirus retinitis in patients with AIDS, as well as patients who have undergone organ transplants, but it has a long history of off-label use. While there are numerous smaller studies attesting to the efficacy of cidofovir, the most recent Cochrane review found only one high-quality study [21]. They found one randomized control trial of 19 patients who received intralesional cidofovir or placebo in double-blinded fashion at the time of surgical debulking, but there was no evidence of difference between placebo and cidofovir at 12 months. In addition to the questions of efficacy, there is some controversy regarding the use of cidofovir due to the potential for serious side effects, including dysplasia, carcinogenesis, neutropenia, and nephrotoxicity. While there have been retrospective studies attesting to the safety of this drug, these studies did not include systematic serologic testing of patients, and larger, prospective cohorts with long-term follow-up are likely necessary to detect significant differences [22, 23].

Level of evidence	Conclusion
1	There is no significant difference between patients treated with cidofovir and placebo at 12 months [21]

Bevacizumab

Zeitels et al. reported a prospective, partially blinded, placebo-controlled study of the antiangiogenic agent bevacizumab as an adjuvant treatment for RRP [24]. They conducted an open-label study in 20 patients with bilateral disease, all of whom underwent planned KTP laser removal. They then treated the more diseased side with bevacizumab and the other with saline. They found that the side receiving bevacizumab had reduced burden of disease compared to control, with improvements in vocal function measures. While the investigation was open label, the ratings of disease burden were carried out in blinded fashion.

Level of evidence	Conclusion
2	Intralesional bevacizumab reduces burden of RRP compared to control [24]

HPV Vaccination

While vaccination does not on its own prevent or cure an existing HPV infection, it does theoretically induce a favorable immune response, which can help the host clear viral burden. A recent systematic review and meta-analysis included 63 patients from 5 studies and showed that the mean number of surgical procedures per month was significantly reduced after HPV vaccination (0.06 vs. 0.35) and the mean interval between surgical intervention increased from 7.02 months to 34.45 months [25].

Level of evidence	Conclusion
1	Meta-analysis of 5 studies demonstrates reduced number of surgeries and prolonged surgical interval after HPV vaccination [25]

Other Agents

Louw reported a preliminary randomized, double-blinded cross-over trial with 10 pediatric RRP patients testing the effects of conjugated-linoleic acid, which has previously been hypothesized to improve outcomes in viral diseases by enhancing the immune response [26]. Of the 10 initial subjects, 8 completed the trial. She reported that patients with moderately aggressive RRP tended to clear the infection without need for further surgery, while more aggressive cases did recur after the treatment period. Due to the low number of patients enrolled, however, it is difficult to extrapolate these results to general clinical practice.

Photodynamic therapy has been used primarily in the treatment of early glottic cancer and dysplasia, but some groups have tried to apply the technique to RRP. The most recent Cochrane review of evidence only found one study of photodynamic therapy with 23 patients that was felt to be low-quality evidence and at high risk of bias [27]. At present, minimal quality evidence exists to support this therapy.

Indole-3-carbinol (I3C) is a known inhibitor of estrogen metabolism found naturally in cruciferous vegetables such as cauliflower, broccoli, and cabbage. One small series reported partial or complete response of 63% of patients after receiving I3C, but this result was not statistically significant, and there has not been any published follow-up [28].

One small study investigated the use of the COX-2 inhibitor celecoxib, which was found in vitro to reduce HPV transcription, and it was effective in clearing papilloma in three patients. However, no follow-up data have been published to date [29].

More recent research has focused on the role of programmed death-ligand 1 (PD-L1), a protein that is elevated in papilloma compared to control tissue [30]. It has been postulated that overexpression of this protein creates a relatively immunosuppressed environment allowing HPV infection to flourish [31]. This has led to the opening of clinical trials for avelumab, a PD-L1 inhibitor that has shown efficacy at improving RRP burden and reducing surgical intervention frequency in a limited pilot study of 12 patients [32]. Further large-scale tests will be necessary to determine the role of this therapy in treatment of RRP.

Conclusion

RRP is a challenging condition due to its irregular growth patterns and ability to elude detection. Surgical removal remains the primary method for treatment, and this can be done with cold or thermal instruments, depending on preference. While the frequently diffuse nature of this disease would appear to invite systemic adjuvant treatment, some historically recommended therapies, such as interferon and cidofovir, do not have a strong evidence basis. Newer therapies, such as HPV vaccination and intralesional bevacizumab, may carry more promise. Finally, the ongoing, population-scale HPV vaccination occurring in many countries may reduce the incidence of RRP further in the years to come, with the ultimate goal of possible eradication.

References

1. Rady PL, Schnadig VJ, Weiss RL, Hughes TK, Tyring SK. Malignant transformation of recurrent respiratory papillomatosis associated with integrated human papillomavirus type 11 DNA and mutation of p53. Laryngoscope. 1998;108(5):735–40.
2. Derkay CS. Task force on recurrent respiratory papillomas. A preliminary report. Arch Otolaryngol Head Neck Surg. 1995;121(12):1386–91.
3. Chesson HW, Ekwueme DU, Saraiya M, Watson M, Lowy DR, Markowitz LE. Estimates of the annual direct medical costs of the prevention and treatment of disease associated with human papillomavirus in the United States. Vaccine. 2012;30(42):6016–9.
4. Shah K, Kashima H, Polk BF, Shah F, Abbey H, Abramson A. Rarity of cesarean delivery in cases of juvenile-onset respiratory papillomatosis. Obstet Gynecol. 1986;68(6):795–9.
5. Ruiz R, Achlatis S, Verma A, et al. Risk factors for adult-onset recurrent respiratory papillomatosis. Laryngoscope. 2014;124(10):2338–44.
6. Taliercio S, Cespedes M, Born H, et al. Adult-onset recurrent respiratory papillomatosis: a review of disease pathogenesis and implications for patient counseling. JAMA Otolaryngol Head Neck Surg. 2015;141(1):78–83.

7. Bryson PC, Leight WD, Zdanski CJ, Drake AF, Rose AS. High-resolution ultrasound in the evaluation of pediatric recurrent respiratory papillomatosis. Arch Otolaryngol Head Neck Surg. 2009;135(3):250–3.

8. Jackowska J, Klimza H, Winiarski P, Piersiala K, Wierzbicka M. The usefulness of narrow band imaging in the assessment of laryngeal papillomatosis. PLoS One. 2018;13(10):e0205554. Published 2018 Oct 9.

9. Tjon Pian Gi RE, Halmos GB, van Hemel BM, et al. Narrow band imaging is a new technique in visualization of recurrent respiratory papillomatosis. Laryngoscope. 2012;122(8):1826–30.

10. Derkay CS, Hester RP, Burke B, Carron J, Lawson L. Analysis of a staging assessment system for prediction of surgical interval in recurrent respiratory papillomatosis. Int J Pediatr Otorhinolaryngol. 2004;68(12):1493–8.

11. Kupfer RA, Çadalli Tatar E, Barry JO, Allen CT, Merati AL. Anatomic Derkay score is associated with voice handicap in laryngeal papillomatosis in adults. Otolaryngol Head Neck Surg. 2016;154(4):689–92.

12. Pasquale K, Wiatrak B, Woolley A, Lewis L. Microdebrider versus CO2 laser removal of recurrent respiratory papillomas: a prospective analysis. Laryngoscope. 2003;113(1):139–43.

13. McMillan K, Shapshay SM, McGilligan JA, Wang Z, Rebeiz EE. A 585-nanometer pulsed dye laser treatment of laryngeal papillomas: preliminary report. Laryngoscope. 1998;108(7):968–72.

14. Burns JA, Zeitels SM, Akst LM, Broadhurst MS, Hillman RE, Anderson R. 532 nm pulsed potassium-titanyl-phosphate laser treatment of laryngeal papillomatosis under general anesthesia. Laryngoscope. 2007;117(8):1500–4.

15. Franco RA Jr, Zeitels SM, Farinelli WA, Anderson RR. 585-nm pulsed dye laser treatment of glottal papillomatosis. Ann Otol Rhinol Laryngol. 2002;111(6):486–92.

16. Rees CJ, Postma GN, Koufman JA. Cost savings of unsedated office-based laser surgery for laryngeal papillomas. Ann Otol Rhinol Laryngol. 2007;116(1):45–8.

17. Nodarse-Cuní H, Iznaga-Marín N, Viera-Alvarez D, et al. Interferon alpha-2b as adjuvant treatment of recurrent respiratory papillomatosis in Cuba: National Programme (1994–1999 report). J Laryngol Otol. 2004;118(9):681–7.

18. Leventhal BG, Kashima HK, Weck PW, et al. Randomized surgical adjuvant trial of interferon alfa-n1 in recurrent papillomatosis. Arch Otolaryngol Head Neck Surg. 1988;114(10):1163–9.

19. Kashima H, Leventhal B, Clark K, et al. Interferon alfa-n1 (Wellferon) in juvenile onset recurrent respiratory papillomatosis: results of a randomized study in twelve collaborative institutions. Laryngoscope. 1988;98(3):334–40.

20. Healy GB, Gelber RD, Trowbridge AL, Grundfast KM, Ruben RJ, Price KN. Treatment of recurrent respiratory papillomatosis with human leuko-

cyte interferon. Results of a multicenter randomized clinical trial. N Engl J Med. 1988;319(7):401–7.

21. Chadha NK, James A. Adjuvant antiviral therapy for recurrent respiratory papillomatosis. Cochrane Database Syst Rev. 2012;12(12):CD005053. Published 2012 Dec 12.

22. Tjon Pian Gi RE, Ilmarinen T, van den Heuvel ER, et al. Safety of intralesional cidofovir in patients with recurrent respiratory papillomatosis: an international retrospective study on 635 RRP patients. Eur Arch Otorhinolaryngol. 2013;270(5):1679–87.

23. Hoesli RC, Thatcher AL, Hogikyan ND, Kupfer RA. Evaluation of safety of intralesional cidofovir for adjuvant treatment of recurrent respiratory papillomatosis [published online ahead of print, 2020 Jan 2]. JAMA Otolaryngol Head Neck Surg. 2020;146(3):231–6.

24. Zeitels SM, Barbu AM, Landau-Zemer T, et al. Local injection of bevacizumab (Avastin) and angiolytic KTP laser treatment of recurrent respiratory papillomatosis of the vocal folds: a prospective study. Ann Otol Rhinol Laryngol. 2011;120(10):627–34.

25. Rosenberg T, Philipsen BB, Mehlum CS, et al. Therapeutic use of the human papillomavirus vaccine on recurrent respiratory papillomatosis: a systematic review and meta-analysis. J Infect Dis. 2019;219(7):1016–25.

26. Louw L. Effects of conjugated linoleic acid and high oleic acid safflower oil in the treatment of children with HPV-induced laryngeal papillomatosis: a randomized, double-blinded and crossover preliminary study. Lipids Health Dis. 2012;11:136. Published 2012 Oct 12.

27. Lieder A, Khan MK, Lippert BM. Photodynamic therapy for recurrent respiratory papillomatosis. Cochrane Database Syst Rev. 2014;(6):CD009810. Published 2014 Jun 5.

28. Rosen CA, Bryson PC. Indole-3-carbinol for recurrent respiratory papillomatosis: long-term results. J Voice. 2004;18(2):248–53.

29. Lucs AV, Wu R, Mullooly V, Abramson AL, Steinberg BM. Constitutive overexpression of the oncogene Rac1 in the airway of recurrent respiratory papillomatosis patients is a targetable host-susceptibility factor. Mol Med. 2012;18(1):244–9.

30. Hatam LJ, Devoti JA, Rosenthal DW, et al. Immune suppression in premalignant respiratory papillomas: enriched functional CD4+Foxp3+ regulatory T cells and PD-1/PD-L1/L2 expression. Clin Cancer Res. 2012;18(7):1925–35.

31. Ahn J, Bishop JA, Roden RBS, Allen CT, Best SRA. The PD-1 and PD-L1 pathway in recurrent respiratory papillomatosis. Laryngoscope. 2018;128(1):E27–32.

32. Allen CT, Lee S, Norberg SM, et al. Safety and clinical activity of PD-L1 blockade in patients with aggressive recurrent respiratory papillomatosis. J Immunother Cancer. 2019;7(1):119.

Early Glottic Cancer

3

Nupur Kapoor Nerurkar, Gauri Kapre,
and Abhishek Vaidya

Introduction

The incidence of all head and neck malignancies is rising world-wide, with carcinoma of the larynx constituting approximately 1% of all cancers [1]. The glottis is the most frequently involved subsite in this organ, and early presentation to the clinician is common due to the obvious symptom of hoarseness. Glottic cancer responds quite favorably to intervention due to its early presentation, coupled with the low rate of regional and distant metastases.

Rates of laryngeal cancer have been reported as 3.6% for men and 0.5% for women [1].

Smokers have a 10–15 times higher risk of developing laryngeal cancers, heavy smokers being at nearly 30 times the risk [2, 3]. Alcohol intake has also been shown to have a linear relationship

N. K. Nerurkar (✉)
Head- Bombay Hospital Voice and Swallowing Center, Bombay Hospital, Mumbai, India

G. Kapre
Neeti Clinics Pvt Ltd, Department of ENT, Nagpur, Maharashtra, India

A. Vaidya
National Cancer Institute, Department of Head and Neck Surgery, Nagpur, Maharashtra, India

© Springer Nature Switzerland AG 2021
D. E. Rosow, C. M. Ivey (eds.), *Evidence-Based Laryngology*,
https://doi.org/10.1007/978-3-030-58494-8_3

with the risk of developing laryngeal malignancies, and the use of both tobacco and alcohol has a synergistic effect [4, 5]. Environmental exposure to asbestos, polycyclic aromatic hydrocarbons, and textile dust has been implicated as potentially carcinogenic for squamous cell carcinoma of the larynx [6, 7]. The correlation between laryngopharyngeal reflux and laryngeal cancer has also been explored in recent literature [8].

The tumor (T) staging of glottic cancers is displayed in Table 3.1 [9]. "Early" glottic cancers, as defined by Ferlito, would typically indicate a minimally invasive neoplastic disease that does not invade muscle or cartilage [10]. Nevertheless, due to the similarity of presentation and treatment, there is general agreement among clinicians to group Tis, T1, and T2 glottic cancers in the category of "early" glottic cancers [11]. This will be the nomenclature for the purposes of this chapter.

Table 3.1 American Joint Committee on Cancer (AJCC) tumor staging of glottic cancers [9]

Tumor Stage (T)		Description
Tis		Carcinoma in situ
T1		Tumor limited to the vocal folds with or without involvement of the anterior commissure, without impaired vocal fold mobility
	T1a	Tumor limited to one vocal fold
	T1b	Tumor extending to both vocal folds
T2		Tumor extending into the supraglottis and/or subglottis, and/or with impaired vocal fold mobility
T3		Tumor limited to the larynx with vocal fold fixation and/or invasion of the paraglottic space, and/or inner cortex of thyroid cartilage
T4		Moderately advanced and very advanced disease
	T4a	Moderately advanced local disease. Tumor invades through the outer cortex of the thyroid cartilage and/or invades tissues beyond the larynx (e.g., trachea, soft tissues of the neck including deep extrinsic muscles of the tongue, strap muscles, thyroid, or esophagus)
	T4b	Very advanced local disease. Invades prevertebral space, encases carotid artery, or invades mediastinal structures

Diagnosis

Patients with glottic lesions typically present early with complaints of a change in the voice, usually perceived as hoarseness. Complaints of dysphagia are rare in early glottic cancers, except for possible aspiration issues in T2 tumors with impaired vocal fold mobility. Less than 1% of patients present with an enlarged neck node, due to the poor lymphatic drainage of the glottis, which is a factor in favor of good prognosis [12].

Detailed history helps to stratify patients who may have risk factors for malignancy. Use of tobacco and alcohol increases risk dramatically and synergistically. Case-control studies have shown 10- to 20-fold increase in cancer risk among active alcohol and tobacco users [13]. Retrospective studies have also indicated a possible, but inconsistent, role for HPV+ in laryngeal cancer, but certainly support HPV+ as a marker for improved survival [14].

Level of evidence	Conclusion
4	Tobacco and alcohol increase cancer risk among active users [13]
4	HPV may have a possible, but inconsistent, role in laryngeal cancer, but data support HPV+ as a marker for improved survival [14]

Laryngoscopy

White light laryngoscopy, followed by biopsy and histopathology for the diagnosis of malignant glottic lesions, is standard when workup of hoarseness reveals a suspicious lesion.

An important facet of patient triage is the accessibility of timely laryngoscopy for patients with hoarseness. It has been shown that when mirror laryngoscopy was performed at the initial visit to the primary care office, diagnostic delay was significantly decreased in a population of patients eventually diagnosed with laryngeal cancer [15]. This same study showed that diagnostic delay was significantly higher for laryngeal cancer when compared with oropharyngeal cancer, and this delay led to a higher hazard ratio. Often visualization of the larynx is not accomplished immediately upon patient presentation and must be done in a subspecialty location. A prospective study referring 300 patients with hoarseness of at least 4 weeks duration directly from the primary physician to an otolaryngology clinic showed that none of the presumed causes documented by the primary physician were accurate and, by performing early endoscopy, the patients with cancer were diagnosed and treated in a timely fashion [16]. Unfortunately, there was no control group provided for statistical analysis, but this paper emphasized the role for early endoscopy in the diagnosis of laryngeal carcinoma.

Level of evidence	Conclusion
4	Early visualization of the larynx decreases treatment delay for laryngeal cancer [16]

Laryngostroboscopy

The addition of laryngostroboscopy (Fig. 3.1) is instrumental for tumor staging and management planning. One limitation of light laryngoscopy is its inability to assess the mucosal wave of the affected vocal fold. A lesion that does not significantly impact the mucosal wave on videostroboscopy is likely to be limited to the superficial layers of the vocal fold, while complete loss of mucosal wave often indicates infiltration of deeper structures. Alteration in the mucosal wave, even in the absence of a proliferative mass, can alert the clinician to a possible subepithelial malignancy. Retrospective studies have shown correlation between absent mucosal wave and histopathologic diagnosis of invasive carcinoma and carcinoma in situ [17]. Tumor extension into the ante-

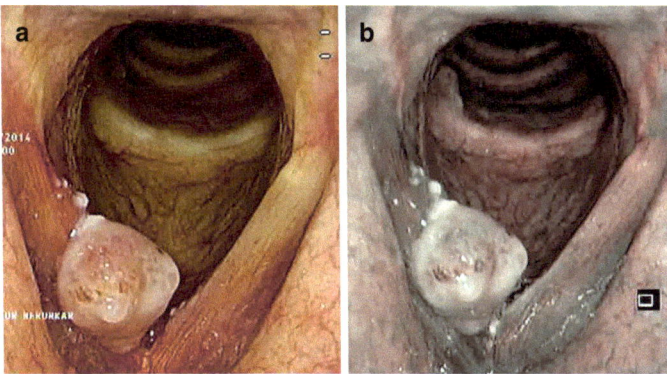

Fig. 3.1 (**a**) Stroboscopic and (**b**) narrow band imaging (NBI) visualization of a right vocal fold lesion concerning for malignancy

rior commissure should be particularly noted to help plan surgical excision if being contemplated. Extension into supraglottic or subglottic tissue should be specifically mapped, as this will upstage the tumor.

Autofluorescence

The fluorescence characteristics of certain tissues are altered during malignant transformation and are able to be measured by exciting the relevant chromophores with light to discern normal from abnormal. Autofluorescence (AF) imaging uses these measurements to differentiate neoplastic changes in the larynx.

A prospective study of 50 patients evaluating the ability of AF and narrow band imaging (NBI) to predict cancer was published in 2016 [18]. Presumptive diagnosis based on each technique was compared with final histopathology after biopsy. It was noted that both AF and NBI showed superior sensitivity when compared with white light endoscopy (WLE). NBI was shown to have better specificity than either WLE or AF.

Narrow Band Imaging

Narrow band imaging (NBI) uses band-filtered light to view vascular proliferation patterns and has been shown to distinguish premalignant and malignant lesions (Fig. 3.1) from benign ones [19]. Ni et al. have proposed a classification for the vascular pattern and the significance of the intraepithelial papillary capillary loop pattern. Types I–IV are considered benign, while type V is considered malignant [20]. An example of type Vb is displayed in Fig. 3.2.

Level of evidence	Conclusion
3	AF and NBI show superior sensitivity to WLE when differentiating premalignant/malignant lesions from benign lesions [18]. NBI showed better specificity than either AF or WLE for differentiating premalignant/malignant lesions from benign lesions [18]

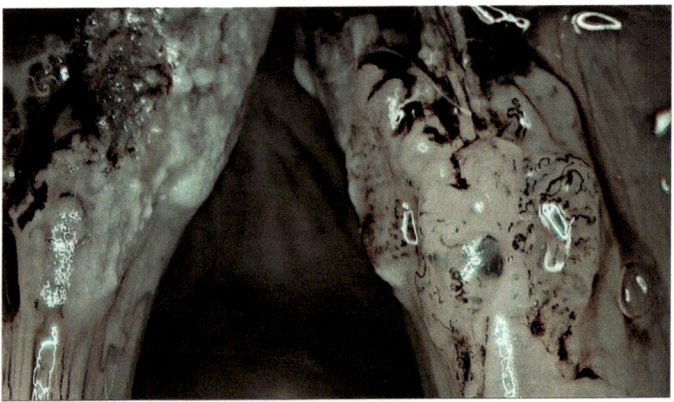

Fig. 3.2 NBI image revealing a Ni type Vb intraepithelial papillary capillary loop pattern on SPIES camera capture in the Spectra A mode suggestive of a malignant lesion. This was confirmed on histopathology in this case

Computed Axial Tomography (CT) and Magnetic Resonance Imaging (MRI)

CT and MRI imaging modalities are useful for evaluating the extent and spread of tumor in the larynx. Invasion of the thyroid cartilage, extension into the anterior commissure, pre-epiglottic or paraglottic space invasion, or any extra-laryngeal spread of the disease needs to be carefully assessed since it has significant implications in treatment planning. In older studies, CT data demonstrated a higher specificity for cartilage invasion than MRI [21]. A more recent prospective, blinded study of CT versus MRI showed very high sensitivity for both modalities, but higher specificity using MRI, especially when assessing disease at the anterior commissure [22]. The authors felt that the addition of diffusion-weighted MRI images (DWI) may have increased the specificity of MRI when compared with older studies. It is also important to consider the expense incurred by the test, the duration of the scan, and patient tolerance, because CT is often favorable for these reasons.

Level of evidence	Conclusion
2	CT and MRI both show high sensitivity for assessment of early glottic cancer, with potential higher specificity for MRI, especially noting disease at the anterior commissure [22]

Positron Emission Tomography (PET)

While PET is not often ordered for diagnosis of early glottic lesions, a recent study assessed whether finding asymmetric FDG-uptake on the vocal folds can be useful in diagnosing tumor [23]. This study retrospectively assessed patients with PET-CT scans showing abnormal fluorodeoxy-D-glucose (FDG) uptake at the larynx or vocal folds and noted in the radiology report. Forty-six patients with positive scans were identified but only 23 of these patients received evaluation by an otolaryngologist. Of the 23 who were not evaluated by an otolaryngologist, 6 had recommendations for referral but were not seen. It was noted that 61 percent of those seen by an otolaryngologist showed true-positive laryngeal disease, while the false-positive rate was 39 percent. While this is level 3 evidence, ENT evaluation for all patients with abnormal FDG uptake at the larynx was recommended, given the false positives outweighed the false negatives.

Histopathologic Diagnosis of Malignancy

Once a patient is suspected of having a malignant laryngeal lesion, histopathological confirmation is necessary. This may be performed as an office procedure or under general anesthesia. For patients who have trismus or a high risk of general anesthesia, a flexible biopsy as an office procedure may be advisable. Care is taken to get a deep enough biopsy to enable comment on invasion of the basement membrane.

Prospective studies have been performed to assess whether in-office biopsies offer the same information as operative biopsy. A 2013 prospective cohort study evaluating patients undergoing in-office biopsy showed an underestimation of disease in approximately 30% of specimens [24]. One partially blinded prospective study showed that in-office biopsy had greater than 80% accuracy rate for determining presence of squamous cell carcinoma (SCC), with a false-positive rate of 0% and a false-negative rate of 18% [25]. Performing in office cytology with biopsy failed to show increased accuracy over biopsy under general anaesthesia alone. The cost of in-office biopsy was significantly less than operative biopsy, and thus the authors recommended in-office biopsy as first step for diagnosis, followed by operative biopsy if negative.

Level of evidence	Conclusion
2	In-office biopsy is more cost effective than operative biopsy [25]

To date, most patients undergo direct laryngoscopic examination and biopsy under general anesthesia. A detailed examination of the extent of the tumor is efficiently performed under magnification with palpation of the lesion, surrounding structures, and arytenoid cartilages to ascertain mobility. If direct laryngoscopy is for the express purpose of diagnostic biopsy then assessment of exposure and access to areas of surgical interest, including the anterior commissure, can be achieved prior to definitive surgery. At times, definitive surgery is planned in the same sitting as initial biopsy, and decisions are made based on frozen section. The reliability of frozen section was quite high in a retrospective study by Remacle et al. where the negative predictive value of frozen section in TLM surgeries was found to be 97% [26]. Most studies have shown an extremely low false-positive rate (0.01%) in frozen histopathology.

Level of evidence	Conclusion
4	Frozen section ability to adequately predict malignancy is high. If frozen section is positive for malignancy, there is an *extremely* low likelihood that final pathology does not support this [26]

Treatment

Treatment options for early glottic cancer include radiotherapy (RT), open laryngeal conservation surgery, and endolaryngeal endoscopic surgery, including transoral laser resection (TLM) [27]. Multiple case series have demonstrated similar survival advantage with these three modalities for T1 and select T2 glottic cancers [28]. A Cochrane systematic review of these modalities was updated in 2014 and noted there were inadequate randomized, prospective studies completed with which to recommend one treatment over another in terms of survival, but RT and endolaryngeal surgery had significant advantages for voice preservation [27]. Multiple meta-analyses have compared endolaryngeal endoscopic resection with RT for early laryngeal cancers and found no significant differences in overall survival or voice outcomes, or evidence favoring any one modality [29–31]. One newer meta-analysis of RT versus TLM has revealed better outcomes with TLM in terms of overall survival, disease specific survival, and organ preservation for T1 glottic disease [32].

The selection of a treatment plan for an individual should be multifactorial. Tumor-related factors, such as T stage, nodal stage, and anatomic extent of disease, are always important, but patient-related factors such as age, profession, general health, and performance status can also help determine the best plan for an individual. Local expertise, for example, renowned TLM surgeons or RT centers that see high volumes, may also be taken into account for best treatment outcomes in a specific region. Appropriate support and rehabilitative services improve outcomes and should be available for best care. An individual patient needs to be made aware of all available factors and options, along with their respective risks and benefits, in order to make an informed decision that makes sense for them. A study by Van Loon et al. showed that 96% of patients preferred TLM to RT [33].

Level of evidence	Conclusions
2/3	Overall there are inadequate randomized, prospective trials to recommend an individual treatment protocol for early glottic cancer. Voice outcomes may be better with RT and endoscopic approaches [27]
2/3	There may be evidence of better outcomes for TLM over RT for overall survival, disease-specific survival, and organ preservation in T1 glottic cancer [32]

Radiation Therapy (RT)

Radiotherapy offers the advantage of a non-surgical intervention with good voice preservation; however, it is a lengthy modality of treatment. RT incurs early toxicity in the form of mucositis and skin reactions and late toxicity in the form of dysphagia and xerostomia, with rarer side effects including laryngeal stenosis and vocal fold paralysis. Radiation has traditionally been the preferred treatment modality for early glottic cancers prior to the adoption of modern transoral laser surgery techniques [27].

Radiotherapy procedure and doses for early glottic carcinoma are briefly highlighted here [34]. The portals used to treat T1N0 and T2N0 glottic carcinomas are limited to the primary lesion due to the low risk of occult nodal metastases in early glottic cancers. Fields are larger for T2 cancers depending on the site and disease extent.

Typical RT doses for T1/T2 lesions are 2.5 Gray (Gy)/fraction for 5 days weekly over 5 weeks for a total dose of 62.5Gy/25 fractions. Patients are treated with cobalt-60 (^{60}Co), 4 megavolt (MV) X-rays, or 6 MV X-rays by linear accelerator. In recent years, patients are increasingly treated with intensity-modulated radiation therapy (IMRT) to reduce doses to surrounding vital structures. There have been extensive numbers of randomized controlled trials to determine whether modifying some of the factors of RT leads to improved outcomes. These studies are beyond the scope of this review, but have been summarized nicely by Yamazaki et al. [35] There are some data indicating that higher MV X-rays do not provide improved survival over ^{60}Co or lower MV treatment. There are also data supporting accelerated fractionation (AF) to decrease the overall treatment time for RT.

Level of evidence	Conclusions
2	High MV X-rays fail to offer better survival over ^{60}Co and low MV X-rays [35]
	AF may decrease overall treatment time for RT while maintaining survival rates [35]

Conservation Laryngeal Surgery

Conservation laryngeal surgeries, also known as open partial laryngectomies, were developed in the 1950s–1960s and remained a viable treatment option for patients who did not want RT or did not have access to RT centers. These procedures still have a role,

Table 3.2 Indications and contraindications for vertical partial laryngectomy (VPL) [37]

Indications for VPL	Contraindications for VPL
Bulky T1 glottic disease	Cricoarytenoid joint involvement
Small T2 glottic lesions	Thyroid cartilage involvement
Early glottic disease with inadequate endoscopic exposure	*Impaired vocal fold mobility due to paraglottic space involvement
Early glottic disease not suited for RT	*Involvement of more than two-thirds of the contralateral vocal fold
Salvage surgery for early glottic disease after RT failure	

Asterisk (*) indicates relative contraindications

albeit limited, for treating bulky T1 or T2 tumors when TLM is technically or oncologically inadequate and when RT is not desired or possible.

Laryngeal conservation surgeries may be defined as procedures that extirpate disease within the larynx while maintaining physiologic speech and swallowing without the need for *permanent* tracheostoma. The goal of these surgeries is to preserve laryngeal function without compromising cure rates. Open partial surgery has been referred to as an "art" in careful patient selection and surgical execution; there is a fine balance between achieving good local control and optimum functional outcomes [36]. These operations are conventionally described in either the vertical or horizontal plane and are termed vertical partial laryngectomy (VPL) and horizontal partial laryngectomy (HPL), respectively. When necessary, procedures may involve resection in both planes. Treatment of early glottic cancer is most often performed in the vertical plane; thus VPLs are more commonly performed. Supracricoid partial laryngectomy may be employed in select cases of T2 glottic cancers. Indications and contraindications for these procedures are listed in Table 3.2 [37].

Endoscopic Laryngeal Surgery

Recent decades have witnessed a growing popularity of endolaryngeal surgery for early glottic cancer. Transoral laser microlaryngeal surgery (TLM) boasts the advantages of shorter hospital stay and shorter duration of treatment, reduced morbidity, avoidance of the side effects of radiation and good vocal outcomes (in limited resections). If the primary treatment was via TLM, the option of radiotherapy is still available to the patient in the event of recurrence. TLM also has lower hidden costs when considering travel time, cost, and loss of man-hours due to absence from work [38].

Extent of endoscopic resection has been classified based on the depth of the surgical resection. The European Laryngological Society (ELS) has proposed a classification of the types of cordectomies which is summarized in Table 3.3 [39]. Figures 3.3 and 3.4 depict examples of type I and type II cordectomies, respectively, for T1 lesions of the vocal fold. When an extensive TLM is performed, as in a type 4 cordectomy or beyond, the voice out-

Table 3.3 Proposed classification of endoscopic cordectomies by the European Laryngological Society (ELS) [39]

Type I	Subepithelial	Removes epithelium and SLP	Spares vocal ligament
Type II	Subligamental	Removes epithelium, SLP, vocal ligament	Spares complete Thyroarytenoid muscle
Type III	Transmuscular	Removes epithelium, SLP, vocal ligament, medial part of thyroarytneoid muscle	Spares lateral part of thyroarytenoid muscle
Type IV	Total/ complete	Removes epithelium, SLP, vocal ligament, complete thyroaryntenoid muscle	Spares inner thyroid perichondrium
Type V	Extended cordectomies		
	a	Includes the opposite vocal fold in the resection	
	b	Includes the ipsilateral arytenoid in the resection	
	c	Includes the ipsilateral ventricular fold in the resection	
	d	Includes up to 1 cm of the subglottis in the resection	
Type VI	Anterior commissurectomy with bilateral anterior cordotomies (added by the ELS in 2007)		
		Removes all vocal fold tissue anteriorly including inner perichondrium of thyroid cartilage and at times ablates portions of anterior thyroid cartilage	

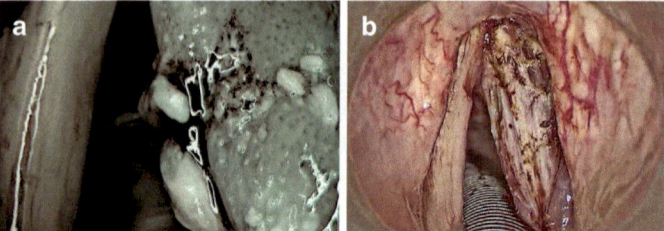

Fig. 3.3 Unilateral right vocal fold lesion before and after European Laryngological Society (ELS) type I resection. (**a**) NBI image revealing a Type 4 Ni pattern with overlying keratotic patches. (**b**) Postoperative picture revealing the exposed vocal ligament following the type I resection

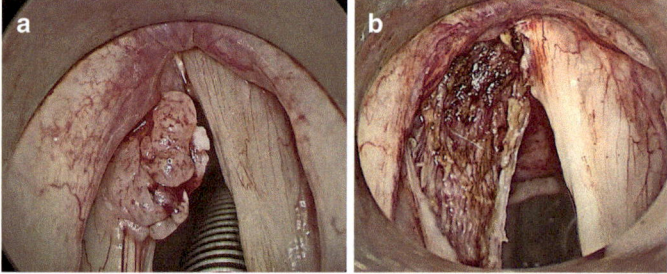

Fig. 3.4 Unilateral left vocal fold lesion before and after ELS type II resection. (**a**) Left vocal fold lesion involving the majority of the vocal fold but sparing the anterior commissure. (**b**) Operative defect where epithelium, superficial lamina propria (SLP), and vocal ligament have been excised. The thyroarytenoid muscle is the deep margin of the excision

comes are quite often very poor, leaving no tissue for medialization laryngoplasty, unless a local flap of tissue is transplanted into the field [40]. An example of a type VI cordectomy is displayed in Fig. 3.5.

Not all glottic cancers will be amenable to transoral microlaryngeal resection. Hence patient selection is of paramount importance. Peretti et al. have given a brief account of a few factors which should be considered for selecting a patient for TLM [41]. Adequate laryngeal exposure is one point which is often underemphasized. There are certain factors that can preoperatively predict a difficult laryngeal exposure such as retrognathia,

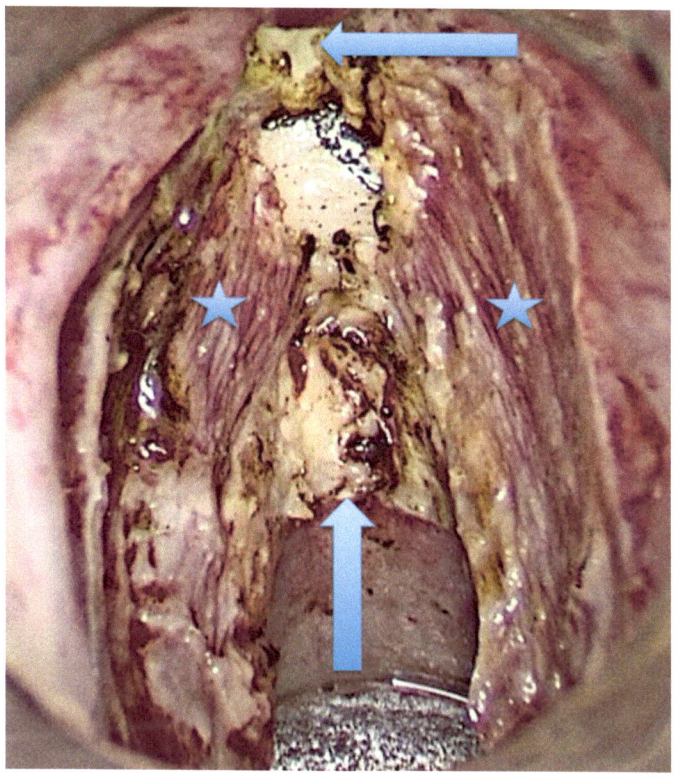

Fig. 3.5 Photograph depicting ELS type VI cordectomy performed with clearance up to the thyroid inner perichondrium from the supraglottis (horizontal arrow) to the subglottis (vertical arrow). The remnant thyroarytenoid muscles are seen bilaterally (stars)

protruding teeth, short neck, obesity, or previously irradiated neck. Laryngeal framework involvement used to be considered an absolute contraindication for TLM; however, Steiner and colleagues have shown that limited resection of the thyroid cartilage can be performed via TLM. Cricoarytenoid joint involvement and arytenoid fixation, involvement of the adjacent muscles, recurrent laryngeal nerve, inferior laryngeal artery, vein and associated lymph channels should also be considered as contraindications for curative resection via TLM [41].

Photodynamic Therapy

Photodynamic therapy is a minimally invasive therapy utilizing a light source to activate light-sensitive drugs, called photosensitizers, into causing tissue destruction [42]. The general principle of PDT is that the light activates the photosensitizer into an excited triplet state. The energy from this excited photosensitizer is then transferred onto the oxygen in the tissue, which gets converted into singlet oxygen which causes tissue destruction by necrosis of cell components. In addition to direct tissue destruction, there is also a release of immune mediators and inflammatory mediators which augment the tissue response. These combined effects lead to tissue destruction within a few days. The extent of tissue destruction depends on the penetration depth of the light source used. The first photosensitizer to be used widely clinically is porfimer sodium (Photofrin), a derivative of hematoporphyrin [43]. The absorption spectrum of porfimer sodium has two significant peaks: the strongest at 400 nm and the weakest at 630 nm. At 400 mm, the depth of penetration of light is less than a millimeter and hence has no clinical application. Hence, 630 nm is used clinically where the light penetrates to a depth of 0.5–1 cm. The light source used for application is usually a pulsed dye laser.

The patient is injected with the photosensitizer drug and is then exposed to the activating light either through the side channel of a flexible laryngoscope or via direct laryngoscopy under general anesthesia. The laser fiber is kept just off the target tissue and light is delivered in a uniform manner. The patient is administered a short course of steroids and analgesics and can usually be discharged the same day. Patients are strongly advised to avoid sun exposure, as this can excite residual photosensitizer in the skin and provoke a significant inflammatory response.

Freche and DeCorbiere have reported a series of early glottic cancers treated with PDT with a 78% complete response for up to 4 years post-treatment [44]. Biel et al. have published the largest group of patients treated with PDT (115 patients) with 91.3% complete response with single treatment [45].

Level of evidence	Conclusions
4	Photodynamic therapy (PDT) may be an alternative treatment for early glottic cancer with good voice preservation [45]

The advantage of PDT is that it can be performed as a single outpatient procedure and may be repeated without significant complications. Post-treatment healing results in normal mucosa and submucosa without notable scarring with resultant good voice preservation [45]. The limitation of PDT is that it can be used only for limited local disease. The photosensitizer may distribute unevenly in the tissue causing suboptimal tissue destruction in some parts of the tumor. It may linger in the skin tissue for prolonged periods making the patient photosensitive for a long time. Commercial availability of suitable photosensitizers is a challenge, which has limited the used of PDT. Until multi-institutional phase II clinical trials substantiate the results of PDT, it will not find a permanent spot in the treatment protocol for laryngeal cancers.

References

1. Bray F, Ferlay J, Soerjomataram I, et al. Global cancer statistics 2018: GLOBOCAN estimates of incidence and mortality worldwide for 36 cancers in 185 countries. CA Cancer J Clin. 2018;68:394–424.
2. Rothman KJ, Cann CI, Flanders D, et al. Epidemiology of laryngeal cancers. Epidemiol Rev. 1980;2:195–209.
3. Kuper H, Boffetta P, Adami HO. Tobacco use and cancer causation: association by tumor type. J Intern Med. 2002;252:206–24.
4. Boffetta P, Hashibe M. Alcohol and cancer. Lancet Oncol. 2003;21:496–505.
5. Bosetti C, Gallus S, Franceschi S, et al. Cancer of the larynx in non smoking alcohol drinkers and in non drinking tobacco smokers. Br J Cancer. 2002;87:516–8.
6. Stell PM, McGill T. Asbestos and laryngeal carcinoma. Lancet. 1973;2:416–7.

7. Paget-Bailley S, Cyr D, Luce D. Occupational exposure and cancer of the larynx- systematic review and meta-analysis. J Occup Environ Med. 2012;54:71–84.

8. Galli J, Camorota G, Volante M, et al. Laryngeal carcinoma and laryngo-pharyngeal reflux disease. Acta Otorhinolaryngol Ital. 2006;26:260–3.

9. American Joint Committee on Cancer. AJCC cancer staging manual. 8th ed; pub Springer international publishing, New York: 2017.

10. Ferlito A, Carbone A, Rinaldo A, et al. "Early" cancer of the larynx: the concept as defined by clinicians, pathologists, and biologists. Ann Otol Rhinol Laryngol. 1996;105(3):245–50.

11. Peretti G, Piazza C, Bolzoni A. Endoscopic treatment for early glottis cancer: indications and oncological outcomes. Otolaryngol Clin North Am. 2006;39:173–89.

12. Landolfo V, Gervasio CF, Riva G, et al. Prognostic role of margin status in open and CO2 laser cordectomy for T1a-b glottis cancer. Braz J Otorhinolaryngol. 2018;84:74–81.

13. Talamini R, Bosetti C, La Vecchia C, et al. Combined effect of tobacco and alcohol on laryngeal cancer risk: a case-control study. Cancer Causes Control. 2002;13(10):957–64.

14. Chen, et al. Clinical impact of human papillomavirus in laryngeal squamous cell carcinoma: a retrospective study. PeerJ. 2017;5:e3395. https://doi.org/10.7717/peerj.3395.

15. Teppo H, Alho OP. Relative importance of diagnostic delays in different head and neck cancers. Clin Otolaryngol. 2008;33:325–30.

16. Hoare T, Thomson H, Proops D. Detection of laryngeal cancer—the case for early specialist assessment. J Royal Soc Med. 1993;86:390–2.

17. Rzepakowska A, Sieska-Badurek E, Osuch-Wojicikiewicz E, et al. The predictive value of videostroboscopy in the assessment of premalignant lesions and early glottis cancers. Ololaryngol Pol. 2017;71(4):14–8.

18. Ni XG, Zhang QQ, Qang GQ. Narrow band imaging versus autofluorescence imaging for head and neck squamous cell carcinoma detection: a prospective study. J Laryngol Otol. 2016;130(11):1001–6.

19. Kimza H, Jackowska J, Wierzbicka M. The usefulness of the NBI- narrow band imaging for the larynx assessment. Otolaryngol Pol. 2018;72(3):1–3.

20. Ni XG, He S, Xu ZG, et al. Endoscopic diagnosis of laryngeal cancer and precancerous lesions by narrow band imaging. J Laryngol Otol. 2011;125(3):288–96.

21. Chu EA, Kim YJ. Laryngeal caner: diagnosis and preoperative workup. Otolaryngol Clin North Am. 2008;42:673–95.

22. Allegra E, Ferrise P, Trapasso S, et al. Early glottic cancer: role of MRI in the preoperative staging. Biomed Res Int. 2014;2014:890385.

23. Seymour N, Burkill G, Harries M. An analysis of true- and false-positive results of vocal fold uptake in positron emission tomography-computed tomography imaging. J Laryngol Otol. 2018;132:270–4.

24. Cohen JT, Safadi A, Fliss DM, et al. Reliability of a transnasal flexible fiberoptic in-office laryngeal biopsy. JAMA Otolaryngol Head Neck Surg. 2013;139(4):341–5.
25. Farias CF, Cobeta I, Souviron R, et al. In-office cup biopsy and laryngeal cytology versus operating room biopsy for the diagnosis of pharyngo-laryngeal tumors: efficacy and cost effectiveness. Head Neck. 2015;37:1483–7.
26. Matar N, Remacle M, Nollevaux MC, et al. Reliability of frozen section analysis in transoral laser microsurgery of upper aerodigestive tract advanced malignant tumours. Int J Phonosurg Laryngol. 2011;1(2):44–6.
27. Forastiere AA, Ismaila N, Lewin JS, et al. Use of larynx-preservation strategies in the treatment of laryngeal cancer: American Society of Clinical Oncology clinical practice guideline update. J Clin Oncol. 2018;36(11):1143–69.
28. Warner L, Chudasama J, Kelly CG, et al. Radiotherapy versus open surgery versus endolaryngeal surgery (with or without laser) for early laryngeal squamous cell cancer. Cochrane Database Syst Rev. 2014;(12):CD002027.
29. Abdurehim Y, Hua Z, Yasin Y, et al. Transoral laser surgery versus radiotherapy: systematic review and meta-analysis for treatment options of T1a glottic cancer. Head Neck. 2012;34:23–33.
30. Feng Y, Wang B, Wen S. Laser surgery versus radiotherapy for T1-T2N0 glottic cancer: a metaanalysis. ORL J Otorhinolaryngol Relat Spec. 2011;73:336–42.
31. Yoo J, Lacchetti C, Hammond JA, et al. Role of endolaryngeal surgery (with or without laser) versus radiotherapy in the management of early (T1) glottic cancer: a systematic review. Head Neck. 2014;36:1807–19.
32. Vaculik MF, MacKay CA, Taylor M, et al. Systematic review and meta-analysis of T1 glottic cancer outcomes comparing CO2 transoral laser microsurgery and radiotherapy. J Otolaryngol Head Neck Surg. 2019;48:44.
33. Van Loon Y, Hendriksma M, Langeveld TPM, et al. Treatment preferences in patients with early glottis cancers. Ann Otol Rhinol Laryngol. 2018;127(3):139–45.
34. Parsons JT, Palta JR, Mendenhall WM, et al. Head and neck cancer. In: Levitt SH, Khan FM, Potish RA, et al., editors. Levitt and Tapley's technological basis of radiation therapy: clinical applications, vol. 3. Baltimore: Lippincott Williams & Wilkins; 1999. p. 269–99.
35. Yamazaki H, Suzuki G, Nakamura S, et al. Radiotherapy for laryngeal cancer—technical aspects and alternate fractionation. J Radiat Res. 2017;58(4):495–508.
36. Tufano RP, Stafford EM. Organ preservation surgery for laryngeal cancer. Otolaryngol Clin North Am. 2008;41(4):741–55.
37. Chawla S, Carney AS. Organ preservation surgery for laryngeal cancer. Head Neck Oncol. 2009;1:12.

38. Smith JC, Johnson JT, Cognetti DM, et al. Quality of life, functional outcome and costs of early glottis cancer. Laryngoscope. 2003;113:68–76.
39. Remacle M, Eckel HE, Antonelli A, et al. Endoscopic cordectomies: a proposal for a classification by the working committee, European Laryngological Society. Eur Arch Otorhinolaryngol. 2000;257:227–31.
40. Nerurkar NK, Deshmukh S. Our approach for optimizing vocal outcomes in transoral laser microsurgical resection of early glottis carcinoma. Int J Phonosurg Laryngol. 2016;6(2):68–72.
41. Peretti G, Piazza C, Mora F, et al. Reasonable limits for transoral laser microsurgery in laryngeal cancer. Curr Opin Otolaryngol Head Neck Surg. 2016;24:135–9.
42. Rigual N, Biel M, Thankappan KK, et al. Photodynamic therapy for laryngeal cancers. Otolaryngol Clin Int J. 2010;2(3):195–9.
43. McCaughan JS. Photodynamic therapy: a review. Drugs Aging. 1999;15(1):49–68.
44. Freche C, DeCorbiere S. Use of photodynamic therapy in the treatment of vocal cord carcinoma. J Photochem Photobiol. 1990;6(3):291–6.
45. Biel MA. Photodynamic therapy treatment of early oral and laryngeal cancers. Photochem Photobiol. 2007;83(5):1063–8.

Unilateral Vocal Fold Paralysis and Paresis

4

Keith A. Chadwick and Lucian Sulica

Introduction

Patients with unilateral vocal fold paralysis and paresis represent a heterogeneous group with wide variation in symptom severity, ranging from mild limitations such as vocal fatigue or difficulty with singing voice, to near aphonia, dysphagia, aspiration, and dyspnea. Appropriate evaluation, counseling, and treatment require an in-depth understanding of the pathophysiology of laryngeal neuropathy because each patient is different, and a "one-size-fits-all" approach is not likely to succeed. Because of the heterogeneity of this population, the breadth of treatment options, and patient and physician preferences, standardizing treatment approaches to obtain high-level evidence has been a challenge [1, 2]. Nevertheless, physicians can help guide patients to treatment options that have the highest likelihood for success by familiarizing themselves with the available literature.

K. A. Chadwick · L. Sulica (✉)
The Sean Parker Institute for the Voice, Department of Otolaryngology-Head & Neck Surgery, Weill Cornell Medical College – New York Presbyterian Hospital, New York, NY, USA
e-mail: lus2005@med.cornell.edu

© Springer Nature Switzerland AG 2021
D. E. Rosow, C. M. Ivey (eds.), *Evidence-Based Laryngology*,
https://doi.org/10.1007/978-3-030-58494-8_4

Etiology and Incidence

Etiology

The first task in the management of unilateral vocal fold paralysis is to determine the underlying cause. Sources of nerve injury fall into three broad categories: damage from surgery or other trauma; compromise from a range of medical conditions causing nerve compression or invasion; and dysfunction due to factors yet to be completely identified, termed "idiopathic." The vast majority of cases of laryngeal paralysis are caused by peripheral neuropathy rather than a central nervous system process. Historically, men have been more often affected because of their increased propensity for smoking and thus, thoracic malignancy. The left vocal fold is more often affected (approximately 60% of cases) due to increased vulnerability of the left recurrent laryngeal nerve to disease and surgery as a result of longer length and more profound descent into the thorax [3]. The relative causes of vocal fold paralysis have been well-studied in a series of historical retrospective reviews, and are summarized in Table 4.1.

Iatrogenic injury has increased over time, probably due to the increased number and variety of surgical procedures which place the laryngeal nerves at risk. Malignancy remains an important cause of vocal fold paralysis, although variability in prevalence may reflect various practices and referral patterns. Neurologic and medical conditions (e.g. tuberculosis) have contributed a decreasing proportion of cases as a result of advances in treatment and preventive care. Despite developments in diagnostic techniques, idiopathic vocal fold paralysis continues to resist further characterization. The relationship between idiopathic vocal fold paralysis and infectious disease has long been apparent. Based on serology, cases have been attributed to Lyme borreliosis, herpes zoster, herpes simplex, Epstein-Barr virus, West Nile virus, and influenza. However, there are no studies that clarify mechanism in the large number of cases in which serologies are negative.

Table 4.1 Causes of vocal fold paralysis

Reference	Year	n	Cause (%)						
			Malignancy	Surgical	Nonsurgical trauma	Intubation	Neurologic	Other medical	Idiopathic
Prasad VMN et al. [4]	2017	161	1%	56%	1%	7%	9%	15%	11%
Cantarella G et al. [5]	2017	356	1%	70%	4%	0%	1%	1%	25%
Spataro et al. [6]	2014	938	18%	56%	3%	6%	2%	2%	13%
Takano et al. [7]	2012	797	13%	52%	3%	7%	4%	4%	17%
Ko et al. [8]	2009	161	12%	48%	7%	0%	5%	6%	22%
Rosenthal et al. [9]	2007	435	13%	46%	2%	4%	3%	14%	18%
Lacourreye O et al. [10]	2003	325	7%	75%	1%	0%	2%	2%	12%
Loughran S et al. [11]	2002	77	52%	22%	0%	5%	0%	9%	12%
León X et al. [12]	2001	171	22%	24%	1%	13%	4%	8%	28%
Srirompotong S et al. [13]	2001	90	29%	24%	6%	2%	4%	0%	34%
Havas T et al. [14]	1999	108	5%	40%	4%	2%	7%	9%	33%
Kelchner LN et al. [15]	1999	117	31%	32%	0%	2%	5%	15%	15%
Benninger MS et al. [16]	1998	280	25%	24%	11%	8%	8%	5%	20%
Ramadan HH et al. [17]	1998	98	32%	30%	7%	4%	8%	3%	16%
Terris DJ et al. [18]	1992	84	40%	35%	1%	7%	2%	4%	11%
Yamada M et al. [19]	1983	519	18%	22%	2%	10%	1%	4%	42%
Woodson GE et al. [20]	1981	84	26%	37%	7%	2%	0%	2%	25%

(continued)

Table 4.1 (continued)

Reference	Year	n	Cause (%)						
			Malignancy	Surgical	Nonsurgical trauma	Intubation	Neurologic	Other medical	Idiopathic
Kearsley JH et al. [21]	1981	80	53%	11%		0%	4%	14%	18%
Tucker HM et al. [22]	1980	210	22%	37%		0%	2%	20%	14%
Maisel RH et al. [23]	1974	127	24%	16%	10%	3%	8%	11%	27%
Parnell FW et al. [24]	1970	86	36%	25%	2%	0%	6%	16%	15%
Hagan PJ [25]	1963	97	28%	34%	0%	0%	8%	11%	19%
Cunning DS [26]	1955	262	27%	7%	1%	0%	8%	11%	53%
Clerf LH [27]	1953	293	39%	21%	2%	0%	0%	9%	29%
Suehs OW [28]	1943	210	31%	15%	2%	0%	2%	23%	26%
Work WP [29]	1941	183	14%	39%	0%	0%	10%	15%	23%
Smith AB et al. [30]	1933	173	27%	15%	1%	0%	4%	36%	17%
New GB et al. [31]	1932	282	31%	11%	1%	0%	5%	17%	35%
Overall[a]		6514	20%	39%	3%	4%	3%	8%	23%

Adapted from Sulica and Blitzer, eds. 2006 [3]

[a]Excluding Kearsley JH et al. [21] and Tucker HM et al. [22] (incomplete data for trauma)

Incidence

The several surgical procedures that place the laryngeal nerves at risk are summarized in Table 4.2. Each of these procedures carries a risk of temporary or permanent paralysis. Although robust evidence regarding the incidence of laryngeal paralysis after these procedures is lacking in many cases, retrospective series have provided an overall estimate after certain surgeries. These incidence rates are summarized in Table 4.3. Prospective incidence rates for vocal fold paralysis are difficult to obtain since many of these procedures are performed by surgeons other than otolaryngolo-

Table 4.2 Surgeries and procedures which place laryngeal nerves at risk

Cervical surgery	Thyroidectomy/parathyroidectomy
	Anterior approach to the cervical spine
	Carotid endarterectomy
	Implantation of vagal nerve stimulator
	Cricopharyngeal myotomy/repair of Zenker's diverticulum
Thoracic procedures	Pneumonectomy and pulmonary lobectomy
	Repair of thoracic aortic aneurysm
	Coronary artery bypass graft
	Aortic valve replacement
	Esophageal surgery
	Tracheal surgery
	Mediastinoscopy
	Thymectomy
	Ligation of persistent ductus arteriosus
	Cardiac and pulmonary transplant
Other surgery	Skull base surgery
	Brainstem surgery (or neurosurgery which required brainstem retraction)
Other procedures	Central venous catheterization
	Endotracheal intubation

Adapted from Sulica and Blitzer, eds. 2006 [3]

Table 4.3 Vocal fold paralysis incidence rates after surgery: composite of representative recent series

Surgery type	Paralysis		Overall
	Temporary	Permanent	
Thyroidectomy	1.0–5.1%	0.4–2.9%	1.0–8.6%
Anterior approach to cervical spine	3.0–20.8%	0.3–6.6%	
Carotid endarterectomy	1.0–7.1%	0.2–5.0%	
Pneumonectomy or lobectomy			6.7–31%
Coronary artery bypass graft (CABG)			0.7–1.9%
Esophagectomy			15–45%

Adapted from Sulica and Blitzer, eds. 2006 [3]

gists, and preoperative evaluation of laryngeal function is not routine. Additionally, patients with complaints of hoarseness after surgery may not be referred to an otolaryngologist in a timely manner.

In addition to the above surgical procedures, endotracheal intubation can cause vocal fold immobility [32, 33]. In the vast majority of these cases, the immobility is neural in origin, and not the result of cricoarytenoid joint disruption [34].

Diagnosis and Work-Up

History

A complete evaluation of a patient with unilateral vocal fold paralysis or paresis begins with a comprehensive history. The most common complaint among these patients is hoarseness, ranging from vocal fatigue to breathy dysphonia to obvious, near-total aphonia. Symptoms tend to correlate with the degree of glottic insufficiency [35]. Patients with vocal fold paralysis may also report dysphagia. Dysphagia may be worse in cases of high vagal injury (in which both the superior and recurrent laryngeal nerves are affected) or when other cranial nerve deficits occur as a result of stroke, skull base surgery or extensive neoplastic processes. Patients may describe shortness of breath occurring during phonation or physical activity; this is usually not true dyspnea, but rather air wasting because of poor glottic valving.

The timing of symptom onset is of paramount importance. Careful questioning should result in a detailed history of other medical events occurring around the time of symptom onset. Patients should be queried about surgery potentially placing the laryngeal nerves at risk, intubation, smoking history, prior chest imaging, and antecedent illnesses. Patients should also be questioned about neurologic symptoms, pulmonary symptoms and a history of exposure to neurotoxic agents.

Patient completion of one of several self-rating scales (e.g. the Voice Handicap Index, [36] the Voice Handicap Index-10, [37] or the Voice-Related Quality of Life [38]) can help determine the level of voice-related disability, track patient outcomes and response to treatment, and aid in interpretation of the copious literature in this area.

Level of evidence	Conclusion
3	Case-control studies show VHI-10 and VRQoL are valid tools for measurement of diagnostic and treatment-related response in patient with vocal fold paralysis [37, 38].

Physical Examination

A complete physical examination of the head and neck should be obtained, including careful palpation of the neck for lymphadenopathy and thyroid disease. In addition, a full evaluation of the cranial nerves should be performed systematically, with special attention to the spinal accessory and hypoglossal nerves (which share the jugular foramen with the vagus) and the other branches of the vagus nerve.

Laryngoscopy and Stroboscopy

Evaluation of the larynx itself should be performed across a variety of laryngeal tasks. Flexible transnasal laryngoscopy probably offers a more accurate impression of laryngeal function since rigid laryngoscopy requires tongue traction and limits the range of laryngeal tasks which can be performed. A hypomobile vocal fold may be surprisingly difficult to appreciate; asking the patient to alternate between sustained vowel phonation and sniffing should make any asymmetry more apparent. The examiner should take care not to be misled by small amounts of vocal fold motion, which may be caused by contralateral innervation of the interarytenoid muscle, cricothyroid muscle activity, or passive lateral displacement of the denervated arytenoid by its contralateral counterpart (the "jostle sign"). The position of the paralyzed vocal fold is not topognostic, nor does it carry information about prognosis [39].

Supraglottic compression may represent compensation for underlying glottic insufficiency, and should clue physicians into the possibility of paralysis or paresis. A prospective study found that patients with glottic insufficiency from vocal fold bowing were 17 times more likely to exhibit abnormal muscle tension patterns [40]. Supraglottic hyperfunction may obstruct the view of the vocal folds, and can be relaxed by maneuvers such as humming or sighing.

Although laryngoscopy provides two-dimensional data, examiners should attempt to judge the three-dimensional relationship of one vocal fold to another. Height mismatch is important to identify as medial displacement of the paralyzed vocal fold may not suffice for treatment. Asymmetry of the arytenoids should also be assessed, as a prolapsed arytenoid can be a sign of severe denervation. Height mismatch and arytenoid prolapse are both potential indications for an arytenoid stabilization procedure, described in further detail below. In addition to laryngoscopy, videostroboscopy should be routinely performed in patients with vocal fold paralysis or paresis to adequately assess the closure pattern of the vocal folds. This is especially important in the evaluation of patients with vocal fold paresis, as subtle glottic insufficiency is difficult to appreciate in continuous light. Video recording of laryngoscopic and stroboscopic examinations helps to track disease progression and recovery, as well as to evaluate outcomes after treatment.

Level of evidence	Conclusion
2	Prospective cohort data shows muscle tension dysphonia (MTD) may be a marker of vocal fold paralysis/paresis [40].

Laryngeal Electromyography

Laryngeal electromyography (LEMG) measures the integrity of laryngeal innervation by means of percutaneous needle electrodes placed into the laryngeal musculature. It can provide unambiguous evidence of denervation and reinnervation and differentiate vocal fold paralysis from mechanical immobility. Its utility in predicting prognosis of vocal fold paralysis has been less clear. This results from varying criteria used to define a "good" or "favorable" prognosis. As with many medical tests, restrictive criteria lead to a higher number of false negatives and more lenient criteria lead to a higher number of false positives. A meta-analysis evaluating the use of LEMG for prognosis has shown that LEMG may be a more reliable predictor of poor outcomes [41]. Of the 503 patients included in the meta-analysis, the overall positive predictive value (accurate prediction of non-recovery of motion) was 90.9% and the overall negative predictive value (accurate prediction of recovery of motion) was 55.6%. This is likely because signs of denervation, like fibrillations and fasciculations, are unambiguous, but signs of reinnervation do not always result in functional recovery. The studies included in this meta-analysis are summarized in Table 4.4. Unfortunately, the majority of these studies were retrospective in study design and follow-up was often shorter than 12 months (range 3–39 months from onset), which may exaggerate the positive predictive value and underestimate the negative predictive value. The subject remains open for further investigation and LEMG is not currently considered essential.

Level of evidence	Conclusion
3	Meta-analysis of retrospective data shows LEMG to be useful in predicting poor nerve outcome [41]

Table 4.4 Laryngeal electromyography and accurate prediction rate in vocal fold paralysis of less than 6 months duration

		Accurate prediction rate	
Study	n	PPV	NPV
Hydman et al. 2009 [42]	15	71.4%	100%
Grosheva et al. 2008 [43]	195	97.2%	59.8%
Wang et al. 2008 [44]	45	78.9%	71.4%
Munin et al. 2003 [45]	31	80%	66.7%
Sittel et al. 2001 [46]	111	94.4%	12.8%
Elez et al. 1998 [47]	20	100%	73.3%
Min et al. 1994 [48]	9	80%	50%
Gupta, Bastian 1993 [49]	18	75%	70%
Hirano et al. 1987 [50]	29	83.3%	58.8%
Parnes, Satya-Murti 1985 [51]	18	100%	78.6%
Overall rate	503	90.9%	55.6%

Adapted from Rickert et al. 2012 [41]

Imaging

Radiographic imaging should be obtained in cases of vocal fold paralysis without an obvious cause, primarily to evaluate for malignancy. Imaging of the entire course of the affected laryngeal nerve is compulsory, including the skull base, mediastinum, and pulmonary apex. Some authors have suggested that routine x-ray radiography is adequate to image the chest; however this may not fully assess all areas where thoracic malignancy may lie. In one study of patients with left vocal fold paralysis, 72% of masses in the aortopulmonary window detected by computed tomography (CT) appeared normal on chest x-ray [52]. Therefore, CT from the base of the skull through the arch of the aorta (for left-sided paralysis) or subclavian artery (for right-sided paralysis) is the minimum recommended study for laryngeal paralysis. The diagnostic yield for CT imaging in vocal fold paralysis is high. In a study of 153 patients with unilateral vocal fold paralysis, subsequent CT scan revealed an underlying etiology in 36 (23.5%) patients [53]. Magnetic resonance imaging (MRI) may be a useful adjunct, particularly in cases of vagal paralysis or when other cranial neuropathies are present, as it offers a more reliable means of imaging the base of skull and central nervous system.

There may be some benefit to obtaining repeat imaging in patients with persistent or progressive paralysis. A retrospective review of 270 patients diagnosed with idiopathic vocal fold paralysis with negative imaging at the time of diagnosis found that approximately 3% developed evidence of a potentially causative lesion on subsequent imaging at a mean time of 23.6 months (median 20.0 months) after onset [54]. Imaging obtained when patients developed new or progressive symptoms revealed a causative lesion in 8 of 29 (28%) patients. The diagnostic yield for routine repeat imaging thus appears low, but should be strongly considered when patients have new or worsening symptoms.

Imaging is not necessary when the cause of vocal fold paralysis is obvious, such as in a case of sudden onset of symptoms immediately after surgery placing the laryngeal nerves at risk. Furthermore, patients with mild vocal fold paresis do not routinely undergo imaging. The overall prevalence of paresis in the general population is high and imaging is very unlikely to reveal a causative lesion. In a study of 176 patients with unilateral vocal fold paresis, 60 of 81 patients with idiopathic paresis underwent CT imaging work-up, ultimately leading to a diagnostic yield of 0% [55]. However, these patients should be followed to ensure that their neurologic deficit does not worsen, which could be a sign of a progressive underlying etiology. In this event, imaging should be obtained.

Evaluation of dysphagia complaints with a modified barium swallow study may be important to initiate swallowing strategies to reduce the risk of aspiration and subsequent pulmonary infection. Retrospective case series show that frank aspiration has been noted in 18 to 38% of patients with vocal fold paralysis with complaints of dysphagia [56–58].

Level of evidence	Conclusion
4	CT from skull base to mid-thorax is effective for determining etiology of vocal fold paralysis when no cause is recognized by physical examination [53]

Serology

A survey of American Broncho-Esophagological Association (ABEA) members from 2006 showed that 71% of respondents found serum testing to be at least occasionally necessary, and 6% felt it was always necessary in the evaluation of patients with unilateral vocal fold paralysis of unknown cause [59]. In this study, most respondents ordered rheumatoid factor, Lyme titer, erythrocyte sedimentation rate, and antinuclear antibody. However, in a prior study of 84 patients undergoing evaluation of unilateral vocal fold paralysis, the yield of serologic testing was 0% [18]. Another study of 231 patients with unilateral vocal fold paralysis and paresis found that some conditions were incidentally diagnosed as a result of serologic testing; however, their causal relationship to vocal fold abnormality could not be established [60]. Therefore, serologic testing is likely of little use unless there is clinical suspicion of a specific underlying illness.

Level of evidence	Conclusion
4	There is no conclusive evidence for ordering serological testing in unilateral vocal fold paralysis [18, 59, 60]

Natural History

Understanding the natural history of vocal fold paralysis is essential to treatment planning and efficacy of intervention. A systematic review of 20 published studies representing 117 cases of idiopathic unilateral vocal fold paralysis showed that some recovery of motion (either complete or partial) occurred in 39% (±20%) of patients with complete recovery of motion in 36% (±22%) [61]. Some recovery of voice function occurred in 61% (±22%) of patients, with complete recovery of voice function occurring in 52% (±17%). The systematic review performed in this study highlighted the fact that many studies do not clearly define recovery as either recovery of voice or recovery of motion. This is an important distinction to make when comparing the results of studies of vocal fold paralysis recovery.

A recent retrospective chart review focused on the natural course of recovery of idiopathic unilateral vocal fold paralysis evaluated recovery of both voice function and vocal fold motion [62]. In this study 69% (38 of 55 patients) recovered vocal function. The mean time to recovery was 152.8 (±109.3) days, with no patients recovering vocal function past 13 months from onset. Of patients who recovered voice, only 22.7% also experienced return of motion. This study showed that the likelihood of recovery decreases as time progresses, with the likelihood of recovery of voice function being 52% at 3 months, 37% at 6 months, 29% at 9 months, and 8% at 12 months. Age, gender, laterality, or use of injection augmentation did not significantly affect the ultimate likelihood of recovery of voice.

A similar study evaluated the natural course of recovery of iatrogenic unilateral vocal fold paralysis and showed that 89.5% (102 of 114 patients) ultimately recovered voice function [63]. The mean time to recovery was 181.8 (±109.3) days. Of patients with recovery of voice, 30.8% experienced return of vocal fold motion. Similar to the study on idiopathic vocal fold paralysis, the likelihood of recovery decreases as length of time from onset of symptoms increases. In this cohort, the likelihood of recovery of voice function was 81% at 1 month, 76% at 3 months, 65% at 6 months, 47% at 9 months, and 25% at 12 months. No patients experienced recovery after 15 months from onset. Patients were stratified based on anatomic site of surgery (skull base, carotid artery, neck surgery, thoracic surgery, and intubation), and mean time to recovery was not significantly different among anatomic subsites. It also did not differ significantly between sides, despite the difference in right and left recurrent laryngeal nerve length. Both of these studies were limited in that patients who underwent definitive intervention early were removed from the cohort, therefore potentially overestimating the likelihood of recovery since those with nerve transection were not included.

Another study evaluating all types of vocal fold paralysis also found through statistical probability modeling that the longer a patient has had symptoms, the lower probability of recovery of voice [64]. Also, patients who had earlier recovery of voice were more likely to experience recovery of motion. The authors of this study discussed that awaiting spontaneous recovery of voice after symptom onset is likely too conservative, and that definitive management should be recommended earlier. Physicians should use this information when having a discussion with the patient about the expected course of recovery and the potential need for intervention.

Treatment

The decision to proceed with intervention in unilateral vocal fold paralysis and paresis are guided by concerns regarding morbidity from dysphagia and aspiration, the patient's perception of their vocal handicap, and expectations about the eventual outcome without treatment. Patients with unilateral paralysis, especially of short duration, can simply be observed, particularly if there is no evidence of aspiration, minimal vocal disability or demand, and/ or good functional prognosis.

Acute Management

The acute management of vocal fold paralysis is difficult to study since diagnosis is often delayed. In a retrospective review of 938 patients with unilateral vocal fold paralysis, the majority of patients are not usually seen by an otolaryngologist until 3–4 months after onset of symptoms [6]. Therefore, high-quality evidence for supportive therapies in the acute stage is significantly limited.

Some management options which have shown good efficacy in other peripheral motor neuropathies, such as idiopathic facial paralysis (Bell's palsy), are often extrapolated to unilateral vocal fold paralysis. However, since the cause of these peripheral neuropathies is not known, it is unclear whether these treatments generalize to all idiopathic motor neuropathies. A Cochrane review on idiopathic facial paralysis showed a significant reduction in the risk (relative risk 0.63 [0.50, 0.80]) of incomplete recovery after 6 months when high-dose corticosteroids are prescribed [65]. In the seven studies included in this meta-analysis, treatment was initiated within 5 days of symptom onset, and within 72 hours in most cases. Limited studies on outcomes of vocal fold paralysis show no significant reduction in risk when steroids are used [66]; however, no randomized controlled clinical trials exist to evaluate this effect.

Another Cochrane review evaluating the benefit of antiviral therapy in idiopathic facial paralysis showed a minor reduction in the risk (relative risk 0.61 [0.39, 0.97]) of incomplete recovery at 3–12 months when patients were treated with antivirals in addition to steroids [67]. Again, acute treatment was initiated early, within 7 days or earlier in the majority of cases. Therefore, treatment with antivirals, especially at the time of presentation, is highly unlikely to have a significant effect.

Nimodipine is a calcium channel blocker typically used to treat hypertension and vasospasm which may also exert a neuroprotective effect on injured neurons by an unknown mechanism. A recent meta-analysis evaluated three quantitative studies comparing the rate of recovery of vocal fold motion in patients with vocal fold paralysis in those who received nimodipine versus controls [68]. In these three studies, a total of 56 patients were included in the nimodipine group and 325 patients were included in the control group. Pooled results found an overall odds ratio of 13.73 [6.21,30.38] favoring recovery of vocal fold motion at 3–6 months after recurrent laryngeal nerve injury in those treated with nimodipine. These results may point to nimodipine as a potential treatment for patients presenting with vocal fold paralysis early in their course; however, the three studies in this meta-analysis were retrospective and cases were primarily compared against a historical cohort, and additional study is needed to determine the true efficacy. Additionally, a longer follow-up time is needed to determine if nimodipine results in an overall improvement in outcomes or merely a brisker recovery.

Voice and Swallowing Therapy

Therapeutic intervention by a speech and language pathologist may help the patient cope with symptoms. Voice therapy can help reduce the muscular tension used to produce voice in the face of glottic insufficiency, and may reduce the effort and fatigue associated with phonation. In addition, a skilled voice therapist may offer patients reassurance and insight into their condition. A meta-analysis of different interventions in vocal fold paralysis and paresis after thyroidectomy showed improvements in subjective voice function and voice handicap index when voice therapy was initiated [69]. Other studies have shown improvements in acoustic measures after voice therapy [70, 71]. However, the heterogeneity of available studies, the patient population, and therapeutic techniques make direct comparisons difficult and limit generalizability of study results [72]. There is currently no convincing clinical evidence that voice therapy is useful to affect the course of vocal fold paralysis. Furthermore, in the absence of randomized controlled trials, it is difficult to determine whether the improvement seen in these studies is a result of intervention or the natural tendency to improve that occurs over time.

Swallowing therapy may be a necessary adjunctive treatment, particularly if the patient has complaints of significant dysphagia or signs of aspiration.

Level of evidence	Conclusion
3	Meta-analysis shows voice therapy is effective for voice improvement after iatrogenic vocal fold paralysis, but no evidence that it changes the motion abnormality present [69]

Neuromuscular Electrical Stimulation

Neuromuscular electrical stimulation (NEMS) is used in other medical specialties and physiotherapy to strengthen weakened musculature [73]. Muscular stimulation seems to have a positive effect on both denervated and paretic muscles [74]. It has therefore been proposed as a possible therapeutic intervention for neurogenic muscular weakness in the larynx. A systematic review of NEMS [73] revealed several studies showing some positive findings, particularly when electrical stimulation-supported voice exercise was compared to conventional voice therapy [75, 76]. However the use of this treatment for patients with vocal fold paralysis and paresis is still investigational, and additional studies are needed to confirm its efficacy as well as to establish standard methods and regimens of treatment.

Injection Augmentation

Even when eventual recovery remains a possibility, patients may desire temporary relief of their symptoms. This can be accomplished by injection of absorbable bulking material into the paralyzed vocal fold to reduce the degree of glottic insufficiency. Multiple substances have been used, including various collagen and hyaluronic acid preparations, micronized human dermis, autologous fat, calcium hydroxylapatite, and carboxymethylcellulose-glycerine gel. Patients should be considered for injection augmentation if they have dysphagia, or if they feel handicapped by their vocal disability. As it is generally a temporary remedy, it is usually reserved for those patients in whom recovery may still occur. It is also considered more effective in less severe glottic insufficiency and cannot reliably modify arytenoid position or posterior insufficiency. Injection can be performed via direct laryngoscopy in the operating room or under topical anesthesia in the awake patient in the office either transorally or percutaneously. A recent systematic review compared the efficacy of injections performed under local anesthesia with those performed under general anesthesia [77]. Four comparison studies included a total of 389 patients; 208 undergoing injection under local anesthesia and 181 undergoing injection under general anesthesia. A variety of injectable materials were used, including hyaluronic acid, calcium hydroxylapatite, and micronized AlloDerm®, and follow-up time ranged from 3 weeks to 12 months. All of these studies showed a significant improvement in patient-reported subjective voice measures, and a pooled analysis of the data in the studies found no significant difference between patients injected under local versus general anesthesia. The results of this systematic review are summarized in Table 4.5.

Table 4.5 Voice outcomes for injection laryngoplasty with local versus general anesthesia

Study	Voice assessment tool	n (LA)	n (GA)	Mean change (LA)	Mean change (GA)	p-value
Chandran et al. 2017 [78]	VHI-10	40	33	15.5	13.9	0.43
Zelenik et al. 2017 [79]	VHI-10	17	14	35.0	31.6	0.664
Mathison et al. 2009 [80]	V-RQOL	50	28	25.1	20.8	0.42
Bove et al. 2007 [81]	VHI-10	31	55	6.9	7.27	0.882

Adapted from Ballard et al. 2018 [77]

Durability of results after injection augmentation depends on the success of the injection as well as the material used. Injection is usually regarded as temporary since the abandonment of polytetrafluoroethylene polymer (Polytef, or Teflon) due to well-known adverse tissue response. Fat is the occasional exception, with results that can persist for up to several years [82, 83]. Voice outcomes are comparable to medialization laryngoplasty or injection with other materials [79, 84, 85]. However results can be unpredictable and diminish over time [86–88]. Calcium hydroxylapatite particle paste has been used since the early 2000s, and positive results tend to last 6–12 months or occasionally longer [89, 90]. Other materials such as hyaluronic acid, collagen, and carboxymethylcellulose show durability of results ranging from 1 month to 12 months [91–98]. Since injection augmentation is used in early cases where recovery is more likely, information about duration is likely to be confounded by natural recovery in some patients.

An evolving body of literature suggests that patients who undergo injection augmentation early in the course of paralysis are less likely to need definitive intervention later, possibly due to placement of the vocal fold in a more favorable position that is maintained by reinnervation [99–102]. A meta-analysis pooled the results of these studies, suggesting that patients who did not receive an early injection were four times more likely to undergo medialization laryngoplasty [103]. However, patients undergoing injection augmentation are generally earlier in the course of their vocal fold paralysis than comparison groups, and thus have better outcome potential regardless of intervention. A randomized controlled clinical trial is needed to verify that the observed effect is not merely the result of selection bias.

Vocal fold injection augmentation has several limitations. First, it cannot reliably reposition the arytenoid to adjust for a height discrepancy or a posterior glottal gap. Additionally, it is not an ideal procedure in large glottic gaps, since larger boluses of injectate can negatively affect the vibratory properties of the vocal fold, even when properly injected. Furthermore, most injection substances require overinjection to allow for partial reabsorption, rendering the fine adjustment of vocal fold position virtually impossible.

The procedure is well-tolerated with minimal discomfort which resolves in several days in the majority of patients [104]. However, it is not without its risks. The most significant is superficial injection. If the injectable material enters the superficial layers of the vocal fold, corrective intervention is challenging and can result in temporary or permanent stiffness and decreased pliability of this tissue. In a study of 962 vocal fold injections with calcium hydroxylapatite, only five injections (0.5%) failed and superficial injection occurred in eight cases (0.8%) [105]. Dyspnea requiring hospitalization occurred in five cases (0.5%), with a combined total complication rate of 1.6%. Severe complications such as abscess, inflammatory reaction, pulmonary embolism, stroke, or mortality (resulting from inadvertent intravascular injection of material) are exceedingly rare [106–112].

Level of evidence	Conclusion
3	Systematic review shows efficacy of injection laryngoplasty for voice improvement regardless of whether general anesthesia is used (office vs. operating room) [77]. Systematic review and meta-analysis data suggest that early injection MAY prevent the need for framework surgery for some patients [103]

Framework Surgery

Laryngeal framework surgery is reserved for symptomatic treatment of glottic insufficiency from unilateral paralysis or paresis which is not expected to improve. It is typically recommended in cases in which nerve transection has occurred or which are over 12 months from onset. In its simplest and most common form, framework surgery consists of medialization laryngoplasty, the surgical insertion of an implant into the paraglottic space to displace the paralyzed vocal fold medially. The laryngeal implant can be made of silicone, formed polytetrafluoroethylene (GoreTex), calcium hydroxylapatite, or another biologically inert material. The procedure is usually performed under local anesthetic so that the surgeon can size and position the implant guided by the patient's phonatory function and flexible laryngoscopy. Success has been amply documented. The most common complication is suboptimal voice outcome, typically due to technical factors. Revision rates range from 5.4% to 14% [113–115], and even as high as 33% when adjunctive procedures such as injection augmentation are included [116].

Several studies have identified factors leading to revision. Patients with a larger posterior glottal gap appear to be more likely to fail unless a procedure to address the posterior gap is performed in addition to implant placement [117–119]. Patients with more severe dysphonia and those who are professional vocalists may be predisposed to a poor functional outcome [116], the latter presumably because of their greater functional requirements. Additionally, patients with vagal (as opposed to recurrent nerve) palsy are well-known to be rehabilitation challenges, as the glottic insufficiency addressed by medialization laryngoplasty represents only one aspect of their neurologic dysfunction.

Arytenoid repositioning or stabilization procedures may be added to medialization laryngoplasty when there is a flaccid, poorly supported arytenoid or a posterior gap, configurations which are notoriously difficult to remedy with thyroplasty alone. An arytenoid procedure positions the vocal process more medially, stabilizes the arytenoid cartilage and increases membranous vocal fold tension. It should always be considered in revision cases, very seriously when there is a persistent posterior gap or unstable arytenoid. In the case of significantly atrophic vocal folds, when a large implant can negatively affect the vibratory properties of the operated vocal fold because of poor soft tissue cover, an arytenoid adduction can help reestablish tension of the vocal fold, effectively "lifting" the vibratory fold off of the underlying implant. An arytenoid procedure can help vertically reposition the membranous vocal fold and minimize height mismatch between vocal folds [120]. Although cadaver studies that show that vocal fold height is not automatically restored to a physiologic position by an arytenoid procedure, addition of a posterior suspension suture stabilizes the arytenoid in a less caudal position and corrects anterior "tipping" of the vocal process during phonation [121]. Arytenopexy shifts the body of the arytenoid medially along cricoid facet rather than rotating the cartilage, and in consequence may offer improved posterior closure and prevent anterior posterior foreshortening during phonation [122]. Arytenoid techniques have shown good efficacy compared to medialization laryngoplasty alone in patients who are carefully selected [123–126]. However, there are no studies which directly compare arytenoid adduction/stabilization and arytenopexy. Because arytenoid procedures are more technically challenging and time-consuming, there is a higher incidence of complications. Edema or bleeding into the paraglottic space is more significant after arytenoid procedures, and can cause airway obstruction requiring temporary tracheostomy [115, 127].

A meta-analysis compared results of studies evaluating outcomes of calcium hydroxylapatite injection augmentation versus silicone or silastic laryngoplasty [128]. This analysis pooled results from 24 studies to include a total of 537 patients: 10 studies on injection laryngoplasty with calcium hydroxylapatite (305 patients) and 14 studies on medialization laryngoplasty (232 patients). Significant improvements in subjective and objective measures of voice function in both groups were observed. The mean voice handicap index (VHI) decreased 36.11 (±6.99) points in the injection group and 38.20 (±17.03) points in the laryngoplasty group. Maximum phonation time also improved in both groups, increasing 5.60 (±1.66) seconds in the injection group and increasing 6.23 (±2.59) seconds in the laryngoplasty group. Meta-analysis of these pooled results found no significant differences between the two groups at the time of follow-up. However, the reader should keep in mind that there may still be significant differences in outcomes of injection augmentation and framework surgery that are obscured when analysis is focused on the pre- and posttreatment change, which is comparably large in both groups.

Level of evidence	Conclusion
3	Meta-analysis of retrospective data shows both injection laryngoplasty with CaHA and laryngeal framework surgery to be successful for improvement of voice quality (VHI) and maximum phonatory time (MPT) in patients with unilateral vocal fold paralysis [128]

Reinnervation

Reinnervation of the larynx using nearby nerves, including both the ansa cervicalis and hypoglossal, is a reasonable treatment option [3]. Compelling a solution as it appears, it is subject to the same limitations as spontaneous recovery. In general, reinnervation increases bulk and tone of the paralyzed vocal fold but does not restore physiologic motion. Reinnervation is ideal when the vocal fold is known to be completely denervated, such as in the case of recurrent laryngeal nerve or vagus nerve transection. Whenever a nerve is transected during surgery, the treatment of choice is immediate re-anastamosis or reinnervation. In cases in which the nerve may be intact, the surgeon should be confident that he or she is not depriving the vocal fold of existing neural input by sectioning a partially recovered recurrent nerve to use the distal stump. LEMG may be useful in making this decision. The patient undergoing reinnervation should be counseled that improvement will occur over the long-term (3–4 months) and that he or she may benefit from an interim rehabilitation technique such as injection laryngoplasty.

A randomized controlled clinical trial of 24 patients undergoing either laryngeal reinnervation (ansa cervicalis) or medialization laryngoplasty showed that both groups had improved functional outcome over baseline, though the difference was not significant [129]. However, subgroup analyses of patients undergoing reinnervation procedures showed that patients whose age was less than 52 years had significantly higher functional scores than those aged over 52 years. In a previous study by Tucker, long-term results of medialization with Silastic implant were compared to those of medialization in conjunction with neuromuscular reinnervation, with long-term voice results favoring the combined neuromuscular reinnervation/medialization procedure [130]. A recent meta-analysis of all procedural interventions for unilateral vocal fold paralysis did not show any significant difference in outcomes between treatment arms; results suggested that reinnervation procedures may provide some additional marginal benefit when combined with framework surgery [125]. Again, differences between treatments are likely to be lost given the large change in pre- and posttreatment measures.

Level of evidence	Conclusion
1	Randomized controlled clinical trial showed medialization laryngoplasty and neuromuscular reinnervation both offer improved functional outcome for vocal fold paralysis [129]

Conclusion

Although a large body of evidence exists to guide physicians in the treatment of unilateral vocal fold paralysis and paresis, the vast majority consist of retrospective reviews and prospective studies with less-than-ideal methodology, small sample sizes and heterogeneous cohorts. Physicians treating unilateral vocal fold paralysis and paresis should be well-versed in this literature so that they may educate and guide patients through treatment options. However, each patient is unique, and this information should be used as a general guide to inform each patient's care while respecting and understanding individual needs and characteristics. Future research efforts should look to establish better practice-based guidelines for treatment that are rooted in well-designed, generalizable, and scientifically valid studies.

Bibliography

1. Walton C, Carding P, Flanagan K. Perspectives on voice treatment for unilateral vocal fold paralysis. Curr Opin Otolaryngol Head Neck Surg. 2018;26(3):157–61.
2. Rosen CA, et al. Nomenclature proposal to describe vocal fold motion impairment. Eur Arch Otorhinolaryngol. 2016;273(8):1995–9.
3. Sulica L, Blitzer A. Vocal fold paralysis. 1st ed. Germany: Springer; 2006.
4. Prasad VMN, et al. Unilateral vocal fold immobility: a tertiary hospital's experience over 5 years. Eur Arch Otorhinolaryngol. 2017;274(7):2855–9.
5. Cantarella G, et al. A retrospective evaluation of the etiology of unilateral vocal fold paralysis over the last 25 years. Eur Arch Otorhinolaryngol. 2017;274(1):347–53.
6. Spataro EA, Grindler DJ, Paniello RC. Etiology and time to presentation of unilateral vocal fold paralysis. Otolaryngol Head Neck Surg. 2014;151(2):286–93.
7. Takano S, et al. Single institutional analysis of trends over 45 years in etiology of vocal fold paralysis. Auris Nasus Larynx. 2012;39(6):597–600.
8. Ko HC, et al. Etiologic features in patients with unilateral vocal fold paralysis in Taiwan. Chang Gung Med J. 2009;32(3):290–6.
9. Rosenthal LH, Benninger MS, Deeb RH. Vocal fold immobility: a longitudinal analysis of etiology over 20 years. Laryngoscope. 2007;117(10):1864–70.
10. Laccourreye O, et al. Unilateral laryngeal paralyses: epidemiological data and therapeutic progress. Presse Med. 2003;32(17):781–6.
11. Loughran S, Alves C, MacGregor FB. Current aetiology of unilateral vocal fold paralysis in a teaching hospital in the West of Scotland. J Laryngol Otol. 2002;116(11):907–10.
12. Leon X, et al. Glottic immobility: retrospective study of 229 cases. Acta Otorrinolaringol Esp. 2001;52(6):486–92.
13. Srirompotong S, Sae-Seow P, Srirompotong S. The cause and evaluation of unilateral vocal cord paralysis. J Med Assoc Thail. 2001;84(6):855–8.
14. Havas T, Lowinger D, Priestley J. Unilateral vocal fold paralysis: causes, options and outcomes. Aust N Z J Surg. 1999;69(7):509–13.

15. Kelchner LN, et al. Etiology, pathophysiology, treatment choices, and voice results for unilateral adductor vocal fold paralysis: a 3-year retrospective. J Voice. 1999;13(4):592–601.

16. Benninger MS, Gillen JB, Altman JS. Changing etiology of vocal fold immobility. Laryngoscope. 1998;108(9):1346–50.

17. Ramadan HH, Wax MK, Avery S. Outcome and changing cause of unilateral vocal cord paralysis. Otolaryngol Head Neck Surg. 1998;118(2):199–202.

18. Terris DJ, Arnstein DP, Nguyen HH. Contemporary evaluation of unilateral vocal cord paralysis. Otolaryngol Head Neck Surg. 1992;107(1):84–90.

19. Yamada M, Hirano M, Ohkubo H. Recurrent laryngeal nerve paralysis. A 10-year review of 564 patients. Auris Nasus Larynx. 1983;10 Suppl:S1–15.

20. Woodson GE, Miller RH. The timing of surgical intervention in vocal cord paralysis. Otolaryngol Head Neck Surg. 1981;89(2):264–7.

21. Kearsley JH. Vocal cord paralysis (VCP)--an aetiologic review of 100 cases over 20 years. Aust NZ J Med. 1981;11(6):663–6.

22. Tucker HM. Vocal cord paralysis--1979: etiology and management. Laryngoscope. 1980;90(4):585–90.

23. Maisel RH, Ogura JH. Evaluation and treatment of vocal cord paralysis. Laryngoscope. 1974;84(2):302–16.

24. Parnell FW, Brandenburg JH. Vocal cord paralysis. A review of 100 cases. Laryngoscope. 1970;80(7):1036–45.

25. Hagan PJ. Vocal cord paralysis. Ann Otol Rhinol Laryngol. 1963;72:206–22.

26. Cunning DS. Unilateral vocal cord paralysis. Ann Otol Rhinol Laryngol. 1955;64(2):487–93.

27. Clerf LH. Unilateral vocal cord paralysis. J Am Med Assoc. 1953;151(11):900–3.

28. Suehs OW. Paralysis of the larynx: a study of 270 cases. Texas State J Med. 1943;38:665–71.

29. Work WP. Paralysis and paresis of the vocal cords: a statistical review. Arch Otolaryngol. 1941;34(2):267–80.

30. Smith AB, Lambert VF, Wallace HL. Paralysis of the recurrent laryngeal nerve. A survey of 235 cases. Edinb Med J. 1933;40(7):344–54.

31. New GB, Childrey JH. Paralysis of the vocal cords: a study of two hundred and seventeen medical cases. Arch Otolaryngol. 1932;16(2):143–59.

32. Colton House J, et al. Laryngeal injury from prolonged intubation: a prospective analysis of contributing factors. Laryngoscope. 2011;121(3):596–600.

33. Kikura M, et al. Age and comorbidity as risk factors for vocal cord paralysis associated with tracheal intubation. Br J Anaesth. 2007;98(4):524–30.

34. Goto T, et al. Unilateral vocal fold adductor paralysis after tracheal intubation. Auris Nasus Larynx. 2018;45(1):178–81.

35. Bielamowicz S, et al. Relationship among glottal area, static supraglottic compression, and laryngeal function studies in unilateral vocal fold paresis and paralysis. J Voice. 2004;18(1):138–45.

36. Jacobson BH, et al. The voice handicap index (VHI): development and validation. Am J Speech Lang Pathol. 1997;6:66–70.

37. Rosen CA, et al. Development and validation of the voice handicap index-10. Laryngoscope. 2004;114(9):1549–56.

38. Hogikyan ND, et al. Voice-related quality of life (V-RQOL) following type I thyroplasty for unilateral vocal fold paralysis. J Voice. 2000;14(3):378–86.

39. Menon JK, Nair RM, Priyanka S. Unilateral vocal fold paralysis: can laryngoscopy predict recovery? A prospective study. J Laryngol Otol. 2014;128(12):1095–104.

40. Belafsky PC, et al. Muscle tension dysphonia as a sign of underlying glottal insufficiency. Otolaryngol Head Neck Surg. 2002;127(5):448–51.

41. Rickert SM, et al. Laryngeal electromyography for prognosis of vocal fold palsy: a meta-analysis. Laryngoscope. 2012;122(1):158–61.

42. Hydman J, et al. Diagnosis and prognosis of iatrogenic injury of the recurrent laryngeal nerve. Ann Otol Rhinol Laryngol. 2009;118(7):506–11.

43. Grosheva M, et al. Evaluation of peripheral vocal cord paralysis by electromyography. Laryngoscope. 2008;118(6):987–90.

44. Wang CC, et al. Prognostic indicators of unilateral vocal fold paralysis. Arch Otolaryngol Head Neck Surg. 2008;134(4):380–8.

45. Munin MC, Rosen CA, Zullo T. Utility of laryngeal electromyography in predicting recovery after vocal fold paralysis. Arch Phys Med Rehabil. 2003;84(8):1150–3.

46. Sittel C, et al. Prognostic value of laryngeal electromyography in vocal fold paralysis. Arch Otolaryngol Head Neck Surg. 2001;127(2):155–60.

47. Elez F, Celik M. The value of laryngeal electromyography in vocal cord paralysis. Muscle Nerve. 1998;21(4):552–3.

48. Min YB, et al. A preliminary study of the prognostic role of electromyography in laryngeal paralysis. Otolaryngol Head Neck Surg. 1994;111(6):770–5.

49. Gupta SR, Bastian RW. Use of laryngeal electromyography in prediction of recovery after vocal cord paralysis. Muscle Nerve. 1993;16(9):977–8.

50. Hirano M, et al. Electromyography for laryngeal paralysis. In: Hirano M, Kirchner JA, Bless DM, editors. Neurolaryngology: recent advances. Boston: College Hill; 1987. p. 232–48.

51. Parnes SM, Satya-Murti S. Predictive value of laryngeal electromyography in patients with vocal cord paralysis of neurogenic origin. Laryngoscope. 1985;95(11):1323–6.

52. Glazer HS, et al. Extralaryngeal causes of vocal cord paralysis: CT evaluation. AJR Am J Roentgenol. 1983;141(3):527–31.

53. Kang BC, et al. Usefulness of computed tomography in the etiologic evaluation of adult unilateral vocal fold paralysis. World J Surg. 2013;37(6):1236–40.

54. Noel JE, Jeffery CC, Damrose E. Repeat imaging in idiopathic unilateral vocal fold paralysis: is it necessary? Ann Otol Rhinol Laryngol. 2016;125(12):1010–4.

55. Badia PI, et al. Computed tomography has low yield in the evaluation of idiopathic unilateral true vocal fold paresis. Laryngoscope. 2013;123(1):204–7.
56. Tabaee A, et al. Flexible endoscopic evaluation of swallowing with sensory testing in patients with unilateral vocal fold immobility: incidence and pathophysiology of aspiration. Laryngoscope. 2005;115(4):565–9.
57. Bhattacharyya N, Kotz T, Shapiro J. Dysphagia and aspiration with unilateral vocal cord immobility: incidence, characterization, and response to surgical treatment. Ann Otol Rhinol Laryngol. 2002;111(8):672–9.
58. Heitmiller RF, Tseng E, Jones B. Prevalence of aspiration and laryngeal penetration in patients with unilateral vocal fold motion impairment. Dysphagia. 2000;15(4):184–7.
59. Merati AL, Halum SL, Smith TL. Diagnostic testing for vocal fold paralysis: survey of practice and evidence-based medicine review. Laryngoscope. 2006;116(9):1539–52.
60. White M, et al. Laboratory evaluation of vocal fold paralysis and paresis. J Voice. 2017;31(2):168–74.
61. Sulica L. The natural history of idiopathic unilateral vocal fold paralysis: evidence and problems. Laryngoscope. 2008;118(7):1303–7.
62. Husain S, et al. Time course of recovery of idiopathic vocal fold paralysis. Laryngoscope. 2018;128(1):148–52.
63. Husain S, et al. Time course of recovery of iatrogenic vocal fold paralysis. Laryngoscope. 2019;129(5):1159–63.
64. Mau T, Pan HM, Childs LF. The natural history of recoverable vocal fold paralysis: implications for kinetics of reinnervation. Laryngoscope. 2017;127(11):2585–90.
65. Madhok VB, et al. Corticosteroids for Bell's palsy (idiopathic facial paralysis). Cochrane Database Syst Rev. 2016;(7):CD001942.
66. Masroor F, et al. The incidence and recovery rate of idiopathic vocal fold paralysis: a population-based study. Eur Arch Otorhinolaryngol. 2019;276(1):153–8.
67. Gagyor I, et al. Antiviral treatment for Bell's palsy (idiopathic facial paralysis). Cochrane Database Syst Rev. 2015;(11):CD001869.
68. Lin RJ, Klein-Fedyshin M, Rosen CA. Nimodipine improves vocal fold and facial motion recovery after injury: a systematic review and meta-analysis. Laryngoscope. 2019;129(4):943–51.
69. Chen X, et al. Types and timing of therapy for vocal fold paresis/paralysis after thyroidectomy: a systematic review and meta-analysis. J Voice. 2014;28(6):799–808.
70. Vij S, Gupta AK, Vir D. Voice quality following unilateral vocal fold paralysis: a randomized comparison of therapeutic modalities. J Voice. 2017;31(6):774 e9–774 e21.
71. Busto-Crespo O, et al. Longitudinal voice outcomes after voice therapy in unilateral vocal fold paralysis. J Voice. 2016;30(6):767 e9–767 e15.
72. Walton C, et al. Unilateral vocal fold paralysis: a systematic review of speech-language pathology management. J Voice. 2017;31(4):509 e7–509 e22.

73. Miller S, et al. Electrical stimulation in treatment of pharyngolaryngeal dysfunctions. Folia Phoniatr Logop. 2013;65(3):154–68.

74. Grill WM, et al. Emerging clinical applications of electrical stimulation: opportunities for restoration of function. J Rehabil Res Dev. 2001;38(6):641–53.

75. Dahl R, Witt G. Analysis of voice parameters after conservative treatment of laryngeal paralysis with conventional voice exercises or neuromuscular electrophonatory stimulation. Folia Phoniatr Logop. 2006;58(6):415–26.

76. Ptok M, Strack D. Electrical stimulation-supported voice exercises are superior to voice exercise therapy alone in patients with unilateral recurrent laryngeal nerve paresis: results from a prospective, randomized clinical trial. Muscle Nerve. 2008;38(2):1005–11.

77. Ballard DP, et al. Systematic review of voice outcomes for injection laryngoplasty performed under local vs general anesthesia. Otolaryngol Head Neck Surg. 2018;159(4):608–14.

78. Chandran D, et al. A comparative study of voice outcomes and complication rates in patients undergoing injection laryngoplasty performed under local versus general anaesthesia: an Adelaide voice specialist's experience. J Laryngol Otol. 2017;131(S1):S41–6.

79. Zelenik K, et al. Comparison of long-term voice outcomes after vocal fold augmentation using autologous fat injection by direct microlaryngoscopy versus office-based calcium hydroxylapatite injection. Eur Arch Otorhinolaryngol. 2017;274(8):3147–51.

80. Mathison CC, et al. Comparison of outcomes and complications between awake and asleep injection laryngoplasty: a case-control study. Laryngoscope. 2009;119(7):1417–23.

81. Bove MJ, et al. Operating room versus office-based injection laryngoplasty: a comparative analysis of reimbursement. Laryngoscope. 2007;117(2):226–30.

82. Pagano R, et al. Long-term results of 18 fat injections in unilateral vocal fold paralysis. J Voice. 2017;31(4):505 e1–9.

83. Umeno H, et al. Analysis of voice function following autologous fat injection for vocal fold paralysis. Otolaryngol Head Neck Surg. 2005;132(1):103–7.

84. Lodder WL, Dikkers FG. Comparison of voice outcome after vocal fold augmentation with fat or calcium hydroxylapatite. Laryngoscope. 2015;125(5):1161–5.

85. Hartl DM, et al. Long-term acoustic comparison of thyroplasty versus autologous fat injection. Ann Otol Rhinol Laryngol. 2009;118(12):827–32.

86. Nishio N, et al. Computed tomographic assessment of autologous fat injection augmentation for vocal fold paralysis. Laryngosc Investig Otolaryngol. 2017;2(6):459–65.

87. Benninger MS, Hanick AL, Nowacki AS. Augmentation autologous adipose injections in the larynx. Ann Otol Rhinol Laryngol. 2016;125(1):25–30.

88. Saccogna PW, et al. Lipoinjection in the paralyzed feline vocal fold: study of graft survival. Otolaryngol Head Neck Surg. 1997;117(5):465–70.

89. Kocdor P, Tulunay-Ugur OE. Injection laryngoplasty outcomes in vocal fold paralysis using calcium hydroxylapatite. Kulak Burun Bogaz Ihtis Derg. 2014;24(5):271–5.

90. Rosen CA, Thekdi AA. Vocal fold augmentation with injectable calcium hydroxylapatite: short-term results. J Voice. 2004;18(3):387–91.

91. Kim YS, et al. Efficiency and durability of hyaluronic acid of different particle sizes as an injectable material for VF augmentation. Acta Otolaryngol. 2015;135(12):1311–8.

92. Miaskiewicz B, et al. Assessment of acoustic characteristics of voice in patients after injection laryngoplasty with hyaluronan. Otolaryngol Pol. 2016;70(1):15–23.

93. Verma SP, Dailey SH. Office-based injection laryngoplasty for the management of unilateral vocal fold paralysis. J Voice. 2014;28(3):382–6.

94. Wen MH, et al. Treatment outcomes of injection laryngoplasty using cross-linked porcine collagen and hyaluronic acid. Otolaryngol Head Neck Surg. 2013;149(6):900–6.

95. Reiter R, Brosch S. Laryngoplasty with hyaluronic acid in patients with unilateral vocal fold paralysis. J Voice. 2012;26(6):785–91.

96. Mallur PS, et al. Safety and efficacy of carboxymethylcellulose in the treatment of glottic insufficiency. Laryngoscope. 2012;122(2):322–6.

97. Arviso LC, et al. Long-term outcomes of injection laryngoplasty in patients with potentially recoverable vocal fold paralysis. Laryngoscope. 2010;120(11):2237–40.

98. Milstein CF, et al. Long-term effects of micronized Alloderm injection for unilateral vocal fold paralysis. Laryngoscope. 2005;115(9):1691–6.

99. Friedman AD, et al. Early versus late injection medialization for unilateral vocal cord paralysis. Laryngoscope. 2010;120(10):2042–6.

100. Yung KC, Likhterov I, Courey MS. Effect of temporary vocal fold injection medialization on the rate of permanent medialization laryngoplasty in unilateral vocal fold paralysis patients. Laryngoscope. 2011;121(10):2191–4.

101. Alghonaim Y, et al. Evaluating the timing of injection laryngoplasty for vocal fold paralysis in an attempt to avoid future type 1 thyroplasty. J Otolaryngol Head Neck Surg. 2013;42:24.

102. Francis DO, et al. Effect of injection augmentation on need for framework surgery in unilateral vocal fold paralysis. Laryngoscope. 2016;126(1):128–34.

103. Vila PM, Bhatt NK, Paniello RC. Early-injection laryngoplasty may lower risk of thyroplasty: a systematic review and meta-analysis. Laryngoscope. 2018;128(4):935–40.

104. Crawley BK, et al. Perception and duration of pain after office-based vocal fold injection augmentation. Laryngoscope. 2018;128(4):929–34.

105. Lee, M., D.Y. Lee, and T.K. Kwon, Safety of office-based percutaneous injection laryngoplasty with calcium hydroxylapatite. Laryngoscope. 2019;129(10):2361–5.

106. Enver, N, et al., A very rare complication of hyaluronic acid injection for medialization laryngoplasty: A case with laryngeal abscess. J Voice. 2020;34(5):812.e5–812.e8.

107. Hamdan AL, Khalifee E. Adverse reaction to restylane: a review of 63 cases of injection laryngoplasty. Ear Nose Throat J. 2019;98(4):212–6.

108. Won SJ, Woo SH. Calcium hydroxylapatite pulmonary embolism after percutaneous injection laryngoplasty. Yonsei Med J. 2017;58(6):1245–8.

109. Dominguez LM, Tibbetts KM, Simpson CB. Inflammatory reaction to hyaluronic acid: a newly described complication in vocal fold augmentation. Laryngoscope. 2017;127(2):445–9.

110. Cohen JC, et al. Severe systemic reaction from calcium hydroxylapatite vocal fold filler. Laryngoscope. 2013;123(9):2237–9.

111. Young VN, et al. An unusual complication of vocal fold lipoinjection: case report and review of the literature. Arch Otolaryngol Head Neck Surg. 2012;138(4):418–20.

112. Zapanta PE, Bielamowicz SA. Laryngeal abscess after injection laryngoplasty with micronized AlloDerm. Laryngoscope. 2004;114(9):1522–4.

113. Weinman EC, Maragos NE. Airway compromise in thyroplasty surgery. Laryngoscope. 2000;110(7):1082–5.

114. Maragos NE. Revision thyroplasty. Ann Otol Rhinol Laryngol. 2001;110(12):1087–92.

115. Rosen CA. Complications of phonosurgery: results of a national survey. Laryngoscope. 1998;108(11 Pt 1):1697–703.

116. Anderson TD, Spiegel JR, Sataloff RT. Thyroplasty revisions: frequency and predictive factors. J Voice. 2003;17(3):442–8.

117. Omori K, et al. Quantitative criteria for predicting thyroplasty type I outcome. Laryngoscope. 1996;106(6):689–93.

118. Koufman JA, Postma GN. Revision laryngoplasty. Op Tech Otolaryngol. 1999;10(1):61–5.

119. Woo P, et al. Failed medialization laryngoplasty: management by revision surgery. Otolaryngol Head Neck Surg. 2001;124(6):615–21.

120. Isshiki N, Tanabe M, Sawada M. Arytenoid adduction for unilateral vocal cord paralysis. Arch Otolaryngol. 1978;104(10):555–8.

121. Woodson GE, et al. Arytenoid adduction: controlling vertical position. Ann Otol Rhinol Laryngol. 2000;109(4):360–4.

122. Zeitels SM, Mauri M, Dailey SH. Adduction arytenopexy for vocal fold paralysis: indications and technique. J Laryngol Otol. 2004;118(7):508–16.

123. Zimmermann TM, et al. Voice outcomes following medialization laryngoplasty with and without arytenoid adduction. Laryngoscope. 2019;129(8):1876–81.
124. Chang J, et al. Outcomes of medialization laryngoplasty with and without arytenoid adduction. Laryngoscope. 2017;127(11):2591–5.
125. Siu J, Tam S, Fung K. A comparison of outcomes in interventions for unilateral vocal fold paralysis: a systematic review. Laryngoscope. 2016;126(7):1616–24.
126. Daniero JJ, Garrett CG, Francis DO. Framework surgery for treatment of unilateral vocal fold paralysis. Curr Otorhinolaryngol Rep. 2014;2(2):119–30.
127. Abraham MT, Gonen M, Kraus DH. Complications of type I thyroplasty and arytenoid adduction. Laryngoscope. 2001;111(8):1322–9.
128. Shen T, Damrose EJ, Morzaria S. A meta-analysis of voice outcome comparing calcium hydroxylapatite injection laryngoplasty to silicone thyroplasty. Otolaryngol Head Neck Surg. 2013;148(2):197–208.
129. Paniello RC, et al. Medialization versus reinnervation for unilateral vocal fold paralysis: a multicenter randomized clinical trial. Laryngoscope. 2011;121(10):2172–9.
130. Tucker HM. Long-term preservation of voice improvement following surgical medialization and reinnervation for unilateral vocal fold paralysis. J Voice. 1999;13(2):251–6.

Spasmodic Dysphonia and Vocal Tremor

5

Diana N. Kirke and Andrew Blitzer

Introduction

Spasmodic dysphonia (SD) is a task-specific, focal laryngeal dystonia that predominantly affects speaking. It has a prevalence of 1/100,000; however, it is a condition thought to be underdiagnosed and thus inadequately treated. In a total population study of primary dystonia in Iceland, the prevalence of SD was 5.9/100,000 [1]. The disorder has either a sudden or gradual onset and occurs most commonly in the fourth or fifth decade of life. Women are more likely to be affected than men at a ratio of approximately 4:1 [2]. SD is of uncertain etiology but it is likely to be multifactorial in most patients. In a small proportion of patients, there is clear familial history, with a rate of 12% reported in the largest treatment series thus far [3]. Vocal tremor (VT) is a separate and distinct disorder characterized by involuntary oscillation of the laryngeal and pharyngeal musculature, resulting in a

D. N. Kirke (✉)
Department of Otolaryngology, Head and Neck Surgery,
Icahn School of Medicine at Mount Sinai, New York, NY, USA
e-mail: diana.kirke@mountsinai.org

A. Blitzer
Department of Otolaryngology, Head and Neck Surgery, Columbia
University College of Physicians and Surgeons, New York, NY, USA

© Springer Nature Switzerland AG 2021   73
D. E. Rosow, C. M. Ivey (eds.), *Evidence-Based Laryngology*,
https://doi.org/10.1007/978-3-030-58494-8_5

modulation of pitch and loudness during voice production. Typically, an affected person cannot sustain a vowel for longer than 5 seconds. Given that a patient may live half his or her life with this disease, it is important to consider the great effect on a patient's emotional state, as well as the impact upon both workplace productivity and social interaction [4].

Spasmodic dysphonia consists of several subtypes including adductor, abductor and mixed spasmodic dysphonia. The more common adductor subtype (ADSD) has a strained quality of speech due to involuntary spasms of the adductor laryngeal muscles. The less common abductor subtype (ABSD) presents with slowed vocal fold closure leading to prolonged voiceless consonants and a breathy quality during speaking. Rarely a patient can present with mixed SD, which is a combination of both ADSD and ABSD. In approximately 25% of patients, SD will also coexist with voice tremor (SD + VT) [2, 5].

Overall there are many features of the etiology, pathophysiology, and phenomenology of SD with or without VT (SD+/-VT) that are still poorly understood, and as such, we present an overview of the disorder as well as the current levels of evidence for both nonsurgical and surgical management.

Etiology and Pathophysiology

The etiology of SD is most likely multifactorial, with possible behavioral and environmental factors contributing to onset of symptoms. In a review of 350 patients, 35% perceived that their disorder was related to an inciting event such as stress, upper respiratory infection, pregnancy, or childbirth [6].

Level of evidence	Conclusion
4	Retrospective review shows 35% of patients perceived that their disorder was related to an inciting event [6].

In 12% of patients, there is a clear familial association, as identified by a positive family history of dystonia [7]. A large subset of this group of patients has undergone genetic studies, and genes associated with laryngeal dystonia have been identified. These include *DYT1* (TOR1A;Locus 9q34), *DYT4* (TUBB4;9p13), *DYT6* (THAP1;8p11), and most recently *DYT25* (GNAL;18p11) [7].

Progress has also been made in understanding the neuropathophysiology of SD, and this has been achieved via studies utilizing advanced neuroimaging modalities. In particular, functional MRI (fMRI) studies have consistently found abnormal activity in the primary sensorimotor, premotor, and sensory association cortices during symptomatic speech tasks [8–10]. During asymptomatic tasks, there is ongoing altered activation in the primary sensorimotor cortex that suggests alteration in the underlying brain structure [9]. An earlier diffusion weighted imaging (DWI) study identified white matter changes along the corticobulbar and corticospinal tracts of SD patients and this then guided the brain tissue analysis of one postmortem SD patient [11]. Compared to three postmortem healthy patients, a reduction of axonal density and myelin content in the genu of the internal capsule was found in the SD patient [11]. More recently, a combined analysis of MRI, fMRI, VBM, and cortical thickness was done in order to examine the structure–function relationship in SD patients [10]. In this study, gray matter volume (GMV), cortical thickness, and brain activation increases were seen in the laryngeal primary sensorimotor cortex, inferior frontal gyrus, superior temporal gyrus, middle temporal gyrus, and cerebellum [10]. When patients with SD + VT were examined with fMRI, voxel-based morphometry (VBM), and DWI, additional abnormalities were found in the middle frontal gyrus and cerebellum, suggesting neuropathophysiological differences between SD + VT patients and those with SD only [12].

Level of evidence	Conclusion
2	Multiple fMRI studies suggest altered activation in the primary sensorimotor cortex suggesting an alteration in brain structure in SD patients [8–10, 12].

Diagnosis

In the largest treatment series thus far of over 1400 patients, 82% of patients had adductor symptoms and 17% abductor symptoms [7]. Of these, about 25% had an irregular dystonic tremor related to their symptoms. Diagnosis generally relies on the use of specific voice tasks in order to elicit spasm of the vocal folds [13], but most physicians will also use direct visualization during these tasks via fiberoptic nasal endoscopy.

Level of evidence	Conclusion
2	The diagnosis of SD generally relies on auditory cues, rather than visual cues [13].

In ADSD, phrases that contain voiced vowels — for example, "we eat eggs every Easter," or counting from 80 to 90 — may elicit hyperadduction of the vocal folds with associated voice breaks and strain. On the other hand, in ABSD, phrases that contain voiceless consonants — for example, "Harry's happy hat" or counting from 60 to 70 — may elicit spasm of the true vocal folds in abduction with associated breathy breaks in the voice.

In those with a dystonic tremor component (SD + VT), one sees rapid, irregular but repetitive movement of the larynx, generally with a directional horizontal preponderance. While the phenomenology of SD + VT is still being elucidated, it has been hypothesized that it may be the result of agonist and antagonist activity of the adductor and abductor musculature. It may be challenging to differentiate SD + VT from essential voice tremor (EVT); however, the latter is not task-specific and generally does not respond to sensory tricks [14].

Other, albeit rare, diagnostic subtypes include mixed SD, singer's SD and adductor breathing SD. In the first subtype, the symptoms may periodically switch between ADSD to ABSD and vice versa. In singer's SD the symptoms only occur during singing; however, in some patients, this may progress also to include speaking activity. Finally in adductor breathing SD, adductor spams occur during inspiration resulting in stridor but not hypoxia [7].

Nonsurgical Management

Botulinum Toxin

There is no cure for SD or VT, but the current gold standard of management for SD (both with and without VT) is Botulinum toxin (BoNT) injection to either the adductor or abductor laryngeal musculature depending on the subtype [2, 3, 15]. BoNT is derived from the bacterium *Clostridium botulinum*, which produces eight immunologically distinct toxins that act as potent neuroparalytic agents: A_{1-8}, B_{1-8}, $C_{1,D}$, D_c, E_{1-12}, F_{1-8}, G, and H [16]. BoNT exerts its effect at the neuromuscular junction by inhibiting the release of acetylcholine (ACh), causing a flaccid paralysis. BoNT type A, onabotulinumtoxinA (Botox; Allergan, Irvine, CA), abobotulinumtoxinA (Dysport; Galderma, Fort Worth, TX), or incobotulinumtoxinA (Xeomin; Merz Pharma GmbH, Frankfurt, Germany) are the most commonly used. BoNT type B, rimabotulinumtoxinB (Myobloc; Solstice Neurosciences, San Francisco, CA) is also commercially available for clinical application.

Currently the literature shows that ADSD patients receive the greatest benefit from BoNT, and this has been supported by a double-blinded, controlled study [17]. Furthermore in such patients, BoNT injection into the thyroarytenoid-vocalis muscle complex has been demonstrated to restore the speaking voice to 60–100% of normal function, with a mean effect of 90% [2]. Injections for ABSD are administered to the posterior cricoarytenoid (PCA) muscle, with a return to mean maximal functional performance of 70% of normal [7]. This disparity in improvement seen with BoNT is likely due to the fact that simultaneous bilateral injections cannot be administered in ABSD patients due to possible compromise of the airway, as well as the increased technical difficulty of accessing and injecting the PCA muscle. As such, 30–40% of patients will also be on oral agents and this will be discussed further below.

Level of evidence	Conclusion
1	BoNT is a safe and effective treatment for adductor spasmodic dysphonia [17].

There are some contraindications for use of BoNT, and there is a paucity of data regarding use during pregnancy. As such, the FDA recommendation is to avoid injection in pregnant or lactating patients. Caution is warranted for the management of patients with conditions such as myasthenia gravis, Lambert-Eaton syndrome and motor neuron disease, particularly when large doses of BoNT are required. However, the amount of toxin that enters the circulation after injection is thought to be minute and this theoretical concern should be balanced against the severity of the hyperkinetic symptoms.

The effective treatment dose is generally variable for each patient and for each muscle injected; therefore, injections are individualized [18]. The dose range for ADSD is 0.05–20 units of BoNT, with an average starting dose of 1.0 unit in 0.1 mL per vocal fold [19]. Subsequent doses are varied according to clinical response and adverse effects, but over time the dose range of BoNT appears to be stable in the majority [20]. When EMG guidance is used for injections, they are done using a tuberculin syringe with a 27-gauge monopolar Polytef-coated hollow EMG recording needle. It is thought that EMG guidance has the advantage of controlled administration into the more actively contracting regions of the muscle; however, it has been found in those experienced with injection that there is not a significant difference between whether it is EMG guided or not [21, 22].

Level of evidence	Conclusion
3	In experienced hands there is no difference whether injections are EMG guided or not [22].

ADSD laryngeal injections are commonly performed percutaneously through the cricothyroid membrane and into the thyroarytenoid–vocalis muscle complex (see Fig. 5.1), though individual practitioner preference may vary.

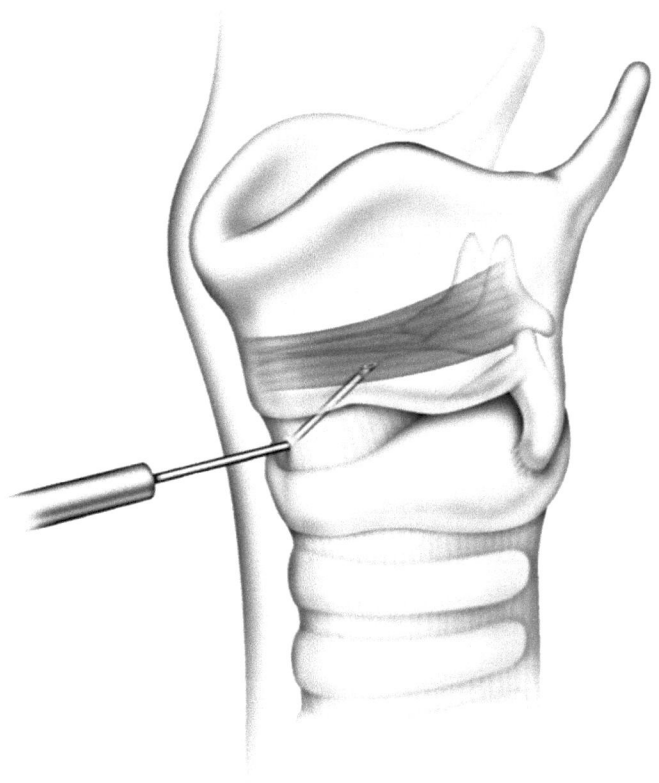

Fig. 5.1 Cricothyroid approach to BoNT injection for adductor spasmodic dysphonia (ADSD)

For ABSD injections, the physician may reach the muscle by manually rotating the larynx, placing the EMG needle behind the posterior edge of the thyroid lamina, and advancing the needle to the cricoid cartilage to arrive at the PCA muscle (see Fig. 5.2). Alternatively, a transcricoid injection can be performed. When the patient is instructed to sniff, thus maximally activating the PCA

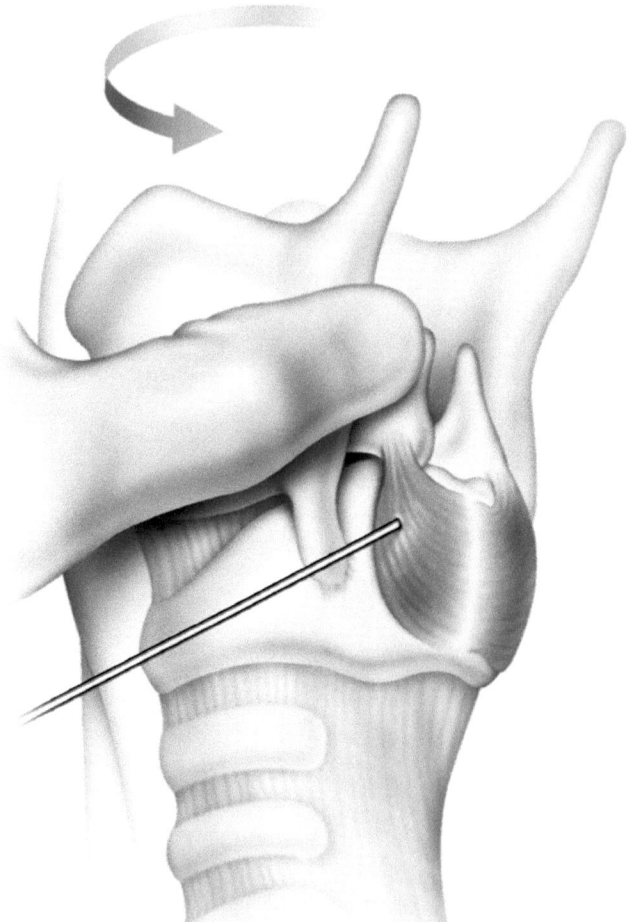

Fig. 5.2 Rotational approach to BoNT injection for abductor spasmodic dysphonia (ABSD)

muscle, a burst of activity is seen on the EMG, and the toxin is administered [23].

Some patients, particularly those with ADSD, may present with excess supraglottic squeeze during the course of their treatment. If these patients are nonresponsive to voice therapy, the supraglottic portion of the lateral cricoarytenoid muscles can be injected via a thyrohyoid approach [24].

The duration of effect of BoNT is between 3 and 4 months and common adverse effects can be separated by subtype. For ADSD they include a mild breathy dysphonia for less than 2 weeks (45%) and mild choking on fluids for the first several days (22%) [7]. For ABSD they include mild stridor and mild dysphagia to solids, the latter being related to diffusion of BoNT to the inferior constrictor muscle. These adverse effects are transient but if the patient has a strong response to therapy and too much weakness occurs they can certainly be counseled that strength and function gradually returns. Follow-up therapy is carefully individualized, and the response to therapy should be meticulously documented.

Voice Therapy

Voice therapy serves purely as an adjunctive, supportive role in the management of SD+/−VT. In a prospective study comparing 10 ADSD subjects treated with BoNT alone, to 17 treated with both BoNT and voice therapy, those treated with combined modality treatment had higher mean airflow rates [25]. The voice therapy treatment in this study was directed at reducing hyperfunctional vocal behaviors and this effect persisted after the voice therapy was complete.

Level of evidence	Conclusion
2	Patients treated with BoNT and voice therapy have higher mean airflow rates, an effect which persists after cessation of voice therapy [25].

Oral Treatments

While the gold standard of treatment for SD is BoNT therapy, there are oral treatments that may play an adjunctive role. Benzodiazepines such as clonazepam or lorazepam are thought to be useful in SD, as GABA has been shown to be deficient in patients with dystonia [26, 27]. As has been previously mentioned, 30–40% of patients with ABSD take benzodiazepines as an adjunctive treatment [7]. Another similar medication is sodium oxybate, which is marketed as Xyrem (Jazz Pharmaceuticals) in the United States and is currently FDA approved for narcolepsy. Its active metabolite, gamma-hydroxybutyric acid (GHB) crosses the blood brain barrier and is converted into gamma-aminobutyric acid (GABA). It then exerts some of its major pharmacologic effects by acting at $GABA_B$ receptors [28]. It has a half-life of 0.5–1 hour, with less than 5% of the drug appearing in urine within 6–8 hours after dosing [29]. Sodium oxybate has been successfully trialled in a single blinded setting in certain alcohol responsive movement disorders, as well as in patients with SD+/-VT [30–33]. Given that the drug has high abuse potential, all patients and their prescribers are enrolled in the Xyrem Risk Evaluation & Mitigation Strategy (REMS) Program formally known as the Xyrem Success Program. This is a central registry that controls the distribution and administration of Xyrem in order to prevent potential abuse and drug diversion [34]. Side effects for this medication noted in all trials included headache, dizziness, and mild sedation. The obvious shortcomings of each of these studies were the administration of Xyrem to patients in an open label fashion and thus the possible placebo effect of the agent; the only clear way to minimize this is via a larger double-blinded randomized controlled trial.

Level of evidence	Conclusion
4	Sodium oxybate may be of benefit in SD with and without VT [32, 33].

In a similar fashion to EVT, the VT component of SD may be adjunctively treated with propranolol and primidone, though this is typically done in conjunction with a movement disorders neurologist.

Surgical Management

SLAD-R

Some patients desire more permanent treatment than is possible with repeat BoNT injections; one surgical alternative for these patients is selective laryngeal adductor denervation – reinnervation (SLAD–R) surgery [35]. In this procedure, the adductor branch of the recurrent laryngeal nerve (RLN) is severed, while the abductor branch is left intact. The adductor branch is then reinnervated with a branch of the ansa cervicalis in order to prevent RLN regrowth, but allows the return of muscle tone and bulk. In a study comparing SLAD–R and BoNT, the former intervention demonstrated statistically significant improved VHI-10 scores pre and post procedure ($p = 0.001$), with these effects persisting at an average of 7.5 years after surgery [35]. However, there was no difference between the two treatments when blinded ratings of voice quality were undertaken. Thus, it is reasonable to conclude that in those experienced with performing SLAD-R, it offers similar outcomes overall to BoNT injection, but higher quality studies are still required to compare the two treatment modalities.

Level of evidence	Conclusion
3	Intervention with SLAD-R demonstrates improved VHI-10 scores compared to BoNT, but no difference on blinded ratings of voice quality between the two treatments [35].

Myectomy

Selective myectomy has been proposed as a possible treatment for both ADSD and ABSD, with the rationale that removal of the dystonic muscle fibers should reduce symptoms. For ADSD, an open thyroarytenoid myectomy can be performed [36–40]. This is undertaken by creating a laryngoplasty window and removing fibers from the thyroarytenoid (TA) and the lateral cricoarytenoid (LCA) muscles until breathiness occurs. Traditionally this open approach is described as a staged procedure with a 3–6 month interval between unilateral procedures [37]. It can also be performed bilaterally via a transoral approach with a CO_2 laser, whereby the mid-posterior bellies of both TA muscles, together with the terminal nerve fibers among deep muscle bundles, are removed [40]. For ABSD, a bilateral endoscopic partial posterior cricoarytenoid (PCA) muscle myoneurectomy has been described, and this is also generally performed as a staged procedure [41]. A CO_2 laser is used to incise along the cricoid cartilage, just lateral to the midline, and the superior aspect of the PCA muscle is divided. In the study that reported this technique, the improvement lasted 8 years postoperatively, as assessed via phone follow-up [41]. No direct comparison has been performed between patients undergoing myectomy and those undergoing BoNT injections, so this category may be considered in patients with disease refractory to BoNT injections.

Level of evidence	Conclusion
4	Multiple case series demonstrate improved voice after selective myectomy for SD.

Type 2 Thyroplasty

The final operative option for patients with ADSD is an Isshiki Type 2 thyroplasty [42]. In this approach, the vocal folds are lateralized in order to prevent tight glottal closure. This is achieved by sectioning the thyroid cartilage in the midline and separating each half permanently with a titanium bridge, without detaching the anterior commissure. This procedure has not been popularized despite long-term follow-up data which show an improvement in voice handicap index-10 (VHI-10) score from 26.3 to 9.4 [43]. Once again, higher quality studies are required to validate the pre-existing research in this area.

Level of evidence	Conclusion
4	Type 2 thyroplasty demonstrates an improvement in VHI-10 scores in SD patients [43].

Conclusion

While much has been learned about diagnosis and treatment of SD+/-VT in recent decades, a great deal remains unknown about these related disorders. There is no question that the use of BoNT is well supported by higher level evidence, while other treatment modalities still require higher quality studies in order to further support their use.

References

1. Asgeirsson H, Jakobsson F, Hjaltason H, Jonsdottir H, Sveinbjornsdottir S. Prevalence study of primary dystonia in Iceland. Mov Disord. 2005;21(3):293–8.
2. Blitzer A, Brin MF, Stewart CF. Botulinum toxin management of spasmodic dysphonia (laryngeal dystonia): a 12-year experience in more than 900 patients. Laryngoscope. 1998;108(10):1435–41.
3. Blitzer A. Spasmodic dysphonia and botulinum toxin: experience from the largest treatment series. Eur J Neurol. 2010;17:28–30.
4. Meyer TK, Hu A, Hillel AD. Voice disorders in the workplace: productivity in spasmodic dysphonia and the impact of botulinum toxin. Laryngoscope. 2013;123:S1–S14.
5. White LJ, Klein AM, Hapner ER, Delgaudio JM, Hanfelt JJ, Jinnah HA, et al. Coprevalence of tremor with spasmodic dysphonia. Laryngoscope. 2011;121(8):1752–5.
6. Childs L, Rickert S, Murry T, Blitzer A, Sulica L. Patient perceptions of factors leading to spasmodic dysphonia: a combined clinical experience of 350 patients. Laryngoscope. 2011;121(10):2195–8.
7. Blitzer A, Brin MF, Simonyan K, Ozelius LJ, Frucht SJ. Phenomenology, genetics, and CNS network abnormalities in laryngeal dystonia: a 30-year experience. Laryngoscope. 2nd ed. 2018;128 Suppl 1(Suppl 1):S1–S9.
8. Haslinger B, Erhard P, Dresel C, Castrop F, Roettinger M, Ceballos-Baumann AO. "Silent event-related" fMRI reveals reduced sensorimotor activation in laryngeal dystonia. Neurology. 2005;65(10):1562–9.

9. Simonyan K, Ludlow CL. Abnormal activation of the primary somato-sensory cortex in spasmodic dysphonia: an fMRI study. Cereb Cortex. 2010;20(11):2749–59.

10. Simonyan K, Ludlow CL. Abnormal structure-function relationship in spasmodic dysphonia. Cereb Cortex. 2012;22(2):417–25.

11. Simonyan K, Tovar-Moll F, Ostuni J, Hallett M, Kalasinsky VF, Lewin-Smith MR, et al. Focal white matter changes in spasmodic dysphonia: a combined diffusion tensor imaging and neuropathological study. Brain. 2007;131(2):447–59.

12. Kirke DN, Battistella G, Kumar V, Rubien-Thomas E, Choy M, Rumbach A, et al. Neural correlates of dystonic tremor: a multimodal study of voice tremor in spasmodic dysphonia. Brain Imaging Behav. 2017;11(1):166–75.

13. Daraei P, Villari CR, Rubin AD, Hillel AT, Hapner ER, Klein AM, et al. The role of laryngoscopy in the diagnosis of spasmodic dysphonia. JAMA Otolaryngol Head Neck Surg. 2014;140(3):228–5.

14. Gurey LE, Sinclair CF, Blitzer A. A new paradigm for the management of essential vocal tremor with botulinum toxin. Laryngoscope. 2013;123:2497–501.

15. Novakovic D, Waters HH, D'Elia JB, Blitzer A. Botulinum toxin treatment of adductor spasmodic dysphonia: longitudinal functional outcomes. Laryngoscope. 2011;121(3):606–12.

16. Peck MW, Smith TJ, Anniballi F, Austin JW, Bano L, Bradshaw M, et al. Historical perspectives and guidelines for botulinum neurotoxin subtype nomenclature. Toxins. 2017;9:38.

17. Troung DD, Rontal M, Rolnick M, Aronson AE, Mistura K. Double-blind controlled study of botulinum toxin in adductor spasmodic dysphonia. Laryngoscope. 1991;101(6 Pt 1):630–4.

18. Meleca RJ, Hogikyan ND, Bastian RW. A comparison of methods of botulinum toxin injection for abductory spasmodic dysphonia. Otolaryngol Head Neck Surg. 1997;117(5):487–92.

19. Blitzer A, Brin MF, Fahn S, Lovelace RE. Localized injections of botulinum toxin for the treatment of focal laryngeal dystonia (spastic dysphonia). Laryngoscope. 1988;98(2):193–7.

20. Tang CG, Novakovic D, Mor N, Blitzer A. Onabotulinum toxin a dosage trends over time for adductor spasmodic dysphonia: a 15-year experience. Laryngoscope. 2016;126(3):678–81.

21. Blitzer A, Lovelace RE, Brin MF, Fahn S, Fink ME. Electromyographic findings in focal laryngeal dystonia (spastic dysphonia). Ann Otol Rhinol Laryngol. 1985;94(6 Pt 1):591–4.

22. Fulmer SL, Merati AL, Blumin JH. Efficacy of laryngeal botulinum toxin injection: comparison of two techniques. Laryngoscope. 2011;121(9):1924–8.

23. Blitzer A, Brin MF, Stewart C, Aviv JE, Fahn S. Abductor laryngeal dystonia: a series treated with botulinum toxin. Laryngoscope. 1992;102(2):163–7.

24. Young N, Blitzer A. Management of supraglottic squeeze in adductor spasmodic dysphonia: a new technique. Laryngoscope. 2007;117(11):2082–4.
25. Murry T, Woodson GE. Combined-modality treatment of adductor spasmodic dysphonia with botulinum toxin and voice therapy. J Voice. 1995;9(4):460–5.
26. Boecker H. Imaging the role of GABA in movement disorders. Curr Neurol Neurosci Rep. 2013;13(10):179.
27. Garibotto V, Romito LM, Elia AE, Soliveri P, Panzacchi A, Carpinelli A, et al. In vivo evidence for GABAA receptor changes in the sensorimotor system in primary dystonia. Mov Disord. 2011;26(5):852–7.
28. Bay T, Eghorn LF, Klein AB, Wellendorph P. GHB receptor targets in the CNS: focus on high-affinity binding sites. Biochem Pharmacol. 2014;87(2):220–8.
29. Xyrem(R) [package insert]. Palo Alto: Jazz Pharmaceuticals, Inc.; 2015.
30. Frucht SJ, Bordelon Y, Houghton WH, Reardan D. A pilot tolerability and efficacy trial of sodium oxybate in ethanol-responsive movement disorders. Mov Disord. 2005;20(10):1330–7.
31. Frucht SJ, Bordelon Y, Houghton WH. Marked amelioration of alcohol-responsive posthypoxic myoclonus by γ-hydroxybutyric acid (Xyrem). Mov Disord. 2005;20(6):745–51.
32. Simonyan K, Frucht SJ. Long-term effect of sodium oxybate (Xyrem®) in spasmodic dysphonia with vocal tremor. Tremor Other Hyperkinet Mov (N Y). 2013;3:tre-03-206-4731-1.
33. Rumbach AF, Blitzer A, Frucht SJ, Simonyan K. An open-label study of sodium oxybate in spasmodic dysphonia. Laryngoscope. 2017;127(6):1402–7.
34. Fuller DE, Hornfeldt CS, Kelloway JS, Stahl PJ, Anderson TF. The Xyrem risk management program. Drug Saf. 2004;27(5):293–306.
35. Mendelsohn AH, Berke GS. Surgery or botulinum toxin for adductor spasmodic dysphonia: a comparative study. Ann Otol Rhinol Laryngol. 2012;121(4):231–8.
36. Genack SH, Woo P, Colton RH, Goyette D. Partial thyroarytenoid myectomy: an animal study investigating a proposed new treatment for adductor spasmodic dysphonia. Otolaryngol Head Neck Surg. 1993;108(3):256–64.
37. Koufman JA, Rees CJ, Halum SL, Blalock D. Treatment of adductor-type spasmodic dysphonia by surgical myectomy: a preliminary report. Ann Otol Rhinol Laryngol. 2006;115(2):97–102.
38. Nakamura K, Muta H, Watanabe Y, Mochizuki R, Yoshida T, Suzuki M. Surgical treatment for adductor spasmodic dysphonia–efficacy of bilateral thyroarytenoid myectomy under microlaryngoscopy. Acta Otolaryngol. 2008;128(12):1348–53.
39. Tsuji DH, Chrispim FS, Imamura R, Sennes LU, Hachiya A. Impact in vocal quality in partial myectomy and neurectomy endoscopic of thyroarytenoid muscle in patients with adductor spasmodic dysphonia. Braz J Otorhinolaryngol. 2006;72(2):261–6.

40. Su C-Y, Chuang H-C, Tsai S-S, Chiu J-F. Transoral approach to laser thyroarytenoid myoneurectomy for treatment of adductor spasmodic dysphonia: short-term results. Ann Otol Rhinol Laryngol. 2007;116(1):11–8.
41. Benito DA, Ferster APO, Sataloff RT. Bilateral posterior cricoarytenoid myoneurectomy for abductor spasmodic dysphonia. J Voice. 2018;34:127.
42. Isshiki N, Haji T, Yamamoto Y, Mahieu HF. Thyroplasty for adductor spasmodic dysphonia: further experiences. Laryngoscope. 2001;111(4 Pt 1):615–21.
43. Sanuki T, Yumoto E. Long-term evaluation of type 2 thyroplasty with titanium bridges for adductor spasmodic dysphonia. Otolaryngol Head Neck Surg. 2017;157(1):80–4.

6

Fermin M. Zubiaur

Introduction

Laryngopharyngeal reflux disease (LPRD) is an inflammatory condition of the upper aerodigestive tract. It is caused by direct and indirect effects of gastroduodenal content reflux which induces morphological changes in the larynx and pharynx [1, 2]. Typical laryngeal symptoms attributed to LPRD include globus pharyngeus, dysphagia, chronic cough, throat clearing, and dysphonia [3]. A vast majority of patients with LPRD have no classic symptoms of gastroesophageal reflux disease (GERD), with only 35 percent reporting heartburn [4]. The ongoing controversy between gastroenterologists and otolaryngologists when diagnosing and treating LPRD supports current medical evidence that GERD and LPRD can be considered and treated as two separate entities.

Differences in the epithelium, and in the physiology between the esophagus and the hypopharynx/larynx, have been well described, including higher sensitivity of the upper aerodigestive

F. M. Zubiaur (✉)
Otorhinolaryngology Surgical Group, Panamericana University School of Medicine, Mexico City, Mexico
e-mail: fzubiaur@clinicadelavoz.com

© Springer Nature Switzerland AG 2021
D. E. Rosow, C. M. Ivey (eds.), *Evidence-Based Laryngology*,
https://doi.org/10.1007/978-3-030-58494-8_6

tract when exposed to caustic chemical injury from pepsin and acid [5]. These differences translate into the need for specific diagnostic methods for GERD vs. LPRD, but current tools lack sensitivity. This leaves a number of symptoms traditionally attributed to LPRD, such as hoarseness, without a clear pathophysiologic mechanism. These limitations in the diagnostic tests available for LPRD limit precise knowledge about its prevalence; nevertheless, LPRD is a common day-to-day diagnosis made by most otolaryngologists. This chapter serves as an overview of the disease and as an updated guide to the current medical evidence available for adequate diagnosis and treatment.

Diagnosis/Pathophysiology

Irritation of the laryngeal mucosa in patients with LPRD can be due to two mechanisms. One mechanism is the effect of gastric contents (acid, pepsin, trypsin, gastroduodenal proteins, and bile salts) directly on the laryngeal mucosa (direct mechanism). The second involves activation of mucosal chemoreceptors by refluxate in the distal esophagus that, in turn, stimulate vagal reflex pathways that cause cough and throat clearing (indirect mechanism) [1].

In the direct mechanism, a number of factors are associated with ongoing chronic laryngeal injury. The laryngeal mucosa in patients with LPRD becomes desensitized, disabling protective mechanisms that would prevent further injury. Study of the adductor reflex response to standardized air-puff stimuli in these patients has suggested that this sensory deficit is improved after 90 days of treatment with an H2 blocker [6].

Pepsin plays an important role in the inflammatory process, as studies have demonstrated its presence in extra- and intracellular laryngeal structures [7–9]. Pepsin may be active at a pH between 1.5 and 6.0, and inactive pepsin molecules in the laryngeal epithelium can persist over time. The reactivation of these proteins is relatively easy in the presence of a moderate gastric reflux episode and/or with the intake of acidic substances. Calvo-Henriquez, et al. performed a systematic review of available studies written on pepsin as a marker of LPR and found that the majority of the papers were able to show a statistically significant difference in pepsin for cases compared with controls [10]. These studies were varied in the assays used for pepsin determination as well as the timing of testing; thus these findings should not be generalized until studies utilizing methodic and consistent testing are available.

Pepsin may act in combination with biliary salts, and the clinician is obligated to consider biliary reflux as a possible cause for resistance to acid suppression therapy. Pepsin can contribute to different types of mucosal injury that are not present in traditional GERD. These mechanisms include depletion of carbonic anhydrase resulting in the over-production of bicarbonate, which decreases cell membrane transepithelial resistance. The reactivation of pepsin in this environment can explain persistent LPRD-related complaints in the presence of weak acidic reflux, and potentially the resistance of symptomatic LPRD patients to traditional empirical treatment for acidic reflux [11, 12].

When LPRD is suspected, dual pH probe studies, despite being the traditional gold-standard for diagnosis, may give negative results and be insufficient to detect the presence of reflux in the laryngopharynx. A hypopharyngeal-esophageal multichannel intraluminal catheter with dual pH (HEMII-pH) test may merit consideration to add diagnostic support in cases of suspected LPRD with negative traditional dual pH probe data [13].

Level of evidence	Conclusion
2	Pepsin testing is able to consistently show cases from control when measured making this a possible marker for diagnosis of LPRD [10].
3	Dual pH probes without proximal esophageal and pharyngeal impedance may be deficient in diagnosing LPRD [13].

Medical Management

PPI Efficacy

Currently, the main treatment strategy for LPRD has been pharmaceutical intervention with Proton Pump Inhibitors (PPIs), accompanied by both lifestyle and dietary changes. The suggested use of PPIs varies among authors but there is a general consensus to prescribe twice-daily PPIs for 3–6 months in order to effectively reduce hypopharyngeal acid reflux [14–16]. A meta-analysis of randomized controlled trials (RCTs) by Liu et al. included a total of 370 patients and suggested that PPIs and placebo therapy were similarly effective in improving LPR symptoms in adult patients [14]. In contrast, another meta-analysis of RCTs by Wei, reporting on 831 patients, concluded that the Reflux Symptom Index (RSI) improved significantly in PPI vs. placebo groups, but response rate (defined as more than 50% reduction in laryngeal symptoms) and Reflux Finding Score (RFS) were not significantly different [15]. A double-blind, placebo controlled trial by Vaezi et al. showed that reduction in RSI and RFS were significantly higher in a group treated with esomeprazole 20 mg twice daily for 3 months over placebo [16]. Many of these studies do not isolate each specific symptom, so the conclusions made just refer to general LPRD symptoms and are based on the validated but still subjective RSI and RFS. As some LPRD-related symptoms such as cough and globus have been more clearly associated, others such as hoarseness have not. To date, the precise mechanisms of voice disorders related to LPRD remain incompletely understood [1]. Lastly, as far as PPIs are concerned, it is important to note that they reduce esophageal acid exposure by changing the chemical nature of refluxate from acid to nonacid, but they do not diminish the total number of reflux episodes [17].

Level of evidence	Conclusion
1	PPIs in one meta-analysis offered no benefit over placebo but in another reduced general LPR symptoms based on the RSI compared to placebo. Response rate and RFS were not significantly different [14, 15].

PPI Side Effects

Proton pump inhibitors are widely prescribed around the world, but important side effects can be associated with them. In addition to unfavorable interactions with certain medications, such as platelet aggregation inhibitors, some studies have shown an increased risk of chronic renal injury, vitamin deficiencies, electrolyte shifts, and an increased risk of myocardial infarction. A prospective cohort study by Gomm et al. showed that in patients 75 years and older, there is an association between PPI use and a new diagnosis of dementia [18]. The use of PPIs in combination with clopidrogrel increases major adverse cardiovascular events in patients with coronary artery disease, but a systematic review found mixed evidence to suggest increased risk of cardiovascular events with PPI monotherapy, independent of clopidrogrel [19]. Another growing concern is the association between PPI use and the risk of fracture and osteoporosis in older women [20, 21]. Numerous observational cohort studies have found an association between PPI use and chronic kidney disease, findings which were confirmed in a recent systematic review and meta-analysis [22]. There is no clear evidence of an increased risk of Alzheimer's disease, specific vascular dementia, or major birth defects with PPI exposure in the first trimester [23, 24].

Level of evidence	Conclusion
2	Chronic use of PPIs is associated with an increased risk of dementia, major cardiac events, osteoporosis, fractures, and chronic kidney disease [18–24].

Other Oral Treatments

Other drugs are commonly used alone or in combination with PPIs for improved acid suppression. H2-receptor antagonists (H2-RAs) are an earlier class of acid-suppression medication. They selectively inhibit the H2 histamine receptor of the parietal cell, leading to suppression of acid secretion. Although they were developed much earlier than PPIs and are very commonly used, they have been found to be significantly less effective than PPIs in controlling GERD symptoms [25].

The potassium competitive acid blockers (P-CABs) have been shown to compete with K^+ and to induce a selective and reversible inhibition of H^+K^+ ATPase in a dose-dependent manner. While PPIs are prodrugs that begin their inhibitory activity after undergoing an acid-catalyzed conversion to a reactive species, P-CABs do not require any molecular rearrangement under acidic conditions, resulting in a more rapid acid suppression. This allows them to elevate intragastric pH to higher levels than PPIs. They are, in fact, able to reach an acid-suppressive effect on the first dose. Vonoprazan is an example of a P-CAB that has been shown to be noninferior to lansoprazole in symptom relief and healing rate in some preliminary trials. However, the possibility of hepatotoxicity associated with P-CABs has limited their routine use in the clinical setting [26].

Prokinetic drugs such as cisapride have been widely used in the past in an attempt to address the pathophysiologic factors resulting in GERD, such as longer clearance time and delayed gastric emptying, but a meta-analysis has shown that this drug is not different from placebo in improving GERD symptoms [25, 27, 28]. Due to adverse side effects from long-term use of cisapride, as well as metoclopramide and domperidone, the popularity of these medications has considerably declined over time, and they are not commonly prescribed. Baclofen, an agonist of GABAb receptors, works in a similar way by inhibiting vagal pathways causing transient lower esophageal sphincter (LES) relaxations. However, its short half-life and frequent side effects make it an unpopular alternative [25, 28].

Anti-depressant drugs, such as tricyclic agents or selective inhibitors of serotonin re-uptake are able to modulate esophageal sensitivity and can be used as adjunctive medications in patients resistant to PPIs, as they have been found to alleviate esophageal discomfort and heartburn. Their known side effects do limit their use, but they can be considered an important alternative if other neurogenic indications are present [25, 29].

There is evidence of altered mucosal integrity in many cases of non-erosive reflux disease which may lead to pain and/or dysmotility. Therefore, pharmacologic interventions that work by directly protecting the esophageal mucosa are an attractive alternative to direct acid suppression. One such compound is sucralfate, which reacts directly with hydrochloric acid to form a thick, protective barrier. Some trials have argued the superiority of sucralfate vs. placebo in alleviating GERD symptoms, and it seems to be equally effective as H2RAs in improving reflux symptoms and in inducing mucosal healing [25, 30]. Alginate is another useful add-on to mainstay treatment, as it has a direct protective effect on esophageal mucosa by the formation of a physical barrier to prevent reflux of gastric contents. A randomized trial shows that the combination of PPIs and alginate was superior to PPIs alone in reducing heartburn symptoms [25, 30–32]. More studies are needed, however, to evaluate the effect of alginates on extra-esophageal and atypical reflux symptoms. Finally, a novel compound consisting of hyaluronic acid and chondroitin sulfate has been recently studied. It works by physical means, coating the esophageal mucosa and acting as a mechanical barrier against acid and pepsin. It has shown promising results in GERD symptom relief with short-term treatment protocols and is intended to be used as an add-on alternative to PPIs [33].

Level of evidence	Conclusion
1	In patients with residual reflux symptoms despite PPI treatment, adding alginate offers additional decrease in the burden of reflux symptoms [31, 32]

Adjuvant Management

Diet/Lifestyle Management

In a retrospective study by Yang et al., an induction program consisting of low-acid/low-fat diet, alkaline water, and behavioral changes, along with anti-reflux medications, demonstrated swift efficacy in ameliorating LPR symptoms compared to a group without dietary changes [34]. Another retrospective study by Zalvan et al. suggests that the effect of PPIs on the reflux symptom index (RSI) is not significantly better than that of alkaline water, a plant-based Mediterranean-style diet, or standard reflux precautions, although the difference in both treatments could be clinically meaningful in favor of the dietary approach [35].

In spite of these findings, the current evidence for dietary recommendations for LPRD mostly originates from retrospective or other low-level evidence. A recent systematic review examining the efficacy of dietary modifications for LPRD treatment suggests that they might improve LPRD symptoms [36]. Nevertheless, the studies that were analyzed in this review, with the exception of a single randomized control trial, were mostly retrospectively designed studies. The authors of the review concluded that there was not sufficient evidence to support dietary recommendations as a primary treatment for LPRD because of the lack of prospective, controlled studies [36].

Level of evidence	Conclusion
4	There is some retrospective data suggesting that dietary modifications may help patients with LPRD symptoms, but there is insufficient prospective evidence to definitively support this [34–36].

There is some evidence, however, that lifestyle changes can be beneficial in reducing LPRD symptoms. A prospective trial of 29 patients, using a standardized behavior modification form, evaluated symptoms for an average of 4 months and found that elevation of the head of bed and avoidance of eating and drinking within 2 hours of sleeping had the most significant influence on LPRD symptoms [37].

Level of evidence	Conclusion
2	Prospective data show that elevation of the head of bed and avoidance of oral intake within 2 hours of lying supine can effectively reduce LPRD symptoms [37].

Upper Esophageal Sphincter Assist Device

A prospective case-control study by Shaker et al., demonstrated that external pressure of 20 to 30 mm Hg applied to the cricoid prevents reflux above the upper esophageal sphincter (UES) by augmenting its intraluminal pressure [38]. The upper esophageal sphincter assist device (UESAD) is applied externally on the neck, it is strapped on with an adjustable band and helps maintain higher UES pressures while it is being worn. Some results so far suggest that the UESAD is an effective noninvasive therapeutic option for reflux-associated laryngeal symptoms and can be considered as an additional therapeutic alternative for LPRD [38, 39].

Level of evidence	Conclusion
3	External cricoid pressure augments the ability of the UES to prevent laryngopharyngeal reflux [38, 39].

Conclusions

A summary of the evidence-based conclusions regarding LPRD may be found in Table 6.1. LPRD is one of the most frequently encountered chronic inflammatory conditions of the upper aerodigestive tract, but its true incidence and prevalence are difficult to estimate because of the lack of consistent and objective diagnostic criteria [40]. Multichannel intraluminal impedance-pH detection is, to date, the most reliable tool for diagnosis even though it is not yet considered gold-standard. It is known that pepsin and bile acids can act as mucosal inflammatory agents, and for this reason, pepsin detection assays should be considered in patients with LPRD symptoms but normal pH probe data.

First-line LPRD treatment combines diet, PPIs, sodium alginate (acid or mixed reflux), and/or anhydrous magaldrate (biliary

Table 6.1 Evidence-based facts for laryngopharyngeal reflux disease

Key concept	Evidence-based fact	Considerations
GERD vs. LPRD	Helpful to approach them as separate diseases	Diagnose and treat individually
LPRD diagnosis	Traditional GERD diagnostic tools do not necessarily diagnose LPRD	Use HEMII-pH when there is unclear diagnosis
Pepsin	Key factor in treatment "failure" or "resistance"	Consider pepsin detection test
Medications	PPIs: mainstay treatment; Alginate and magaldrate: useful add-ons for nonacid reflux	Remember there is limited benefit from using H2 blockers and prokinetics. Keep in mind PPI adverse effects
Diet / lifestyle modifications	Appear to be useful, but not proven in higher-quality studies	Low-risk; consider including as part of comprehensive treatment

LPRD laryngopharyngeal refux disease, *GERD* gastroesophageal reflux disease, *HEMII-pH* hypopharyngeal and esophageal multichannel intraluminal impedance and pH metry, *PPIs* proton pump inhibitors

reflux). Alginate drugs make particular sense in the case of non-acid, mixed reflux, or in patients with postprandial symptoms. The combination of magaldrate after meals and alginate at bedtime may be beneficial for many patients. Dietary and lifestyle modifications show promise in management of symptoms, but more rigorously designed studies are needed to evaluate these modalities.

References

1. Lechien JR, Saussez S, Harmegnies B, Finck C, Burns JA. Laryngopharyngeal reflux and voice disorders: multifactorial model of etiology and pathophysiology. J Voice. 2017;31(6):733–52.

2. Lechien JR, Saussez S, Karkos PD. Laryngopharyngeal reflux disease: clinical presentation, diagnosis and therapeutic challenges in 2018. Curr Opin Otolaryngol Head Neck Surg. 2018;26(6):392–402.

3. Koufman JA. The otolaryngologic manifestations of gastroesophageal reflux disease (GERD): a clinical investigation of 225 patients using ambulatory 24-hour pH monitoring and an experimental investigation of the role of acid and pepsin in the development of laryngeal injury. Laryngoscope. 1991;101:1.

4. Franco RAJ, Deschler DG, Kunins L. Laryngopharyngeal reflux. In Post TW, editor. UpToDate. Waltham: UpToDate Inc.; 2018. Retrieved November 2018, from https://www.uptodate.com/contents/laryngopharyngeal-reflux.

5. Axford SE, Sharp N, Ross PE, et al. Cell biology of laryngeal epithelial defenses in health and disease: preliminary studies. Ann Otol Rhinol Laryngol. 2001;110(12):1099–108.

6. Aviv JE, Liu H, Parides M, Kaplan ST, Close LG. Laryngopharyngeal sensory deficits in patients with laryngopharyngeal reflux and dysphagia. Ann Otol Rhinol Laryngol. 2000;109(11):1000–6.

7. Bulmer DM, Ali MS, Brownlee IA, Dettmar PW, Pearson JP. Laryngeal mucosa: its susceptibility to damage by acid and pepsin. Laryngoscope. 2010;120(4):777–82.

8. Na SY, Kwon OE, Lee YC, Eun YG. Optimal timing of saliva collection to detect pepsin in patients with laryngopharyngeal reflux. Laryngoscope. 2016;126(12):2770–3.

9. Johnston N, Wells CW, Samuels TL, Blumin JH. Pepsin in nonacidic refluxate can damage hypopharyngeal epithelial cells. Ann Otol Rhinol Laryngol. 2009;118(9):677–85.

10. Calvo-Henriquez C, Ruano-Ravina A, Vaamonde P, Martinez-Capoccioni G, amd Martin-Martin C. Is pepsin a reliable marker of laryngopharyngeal reflux? A systematic review. Otolaryngol Head Neck Surg. 2017;157(3):385–91.

11. Johnston N, Knight J, Dettmar PW, Lively MO, Koufman J. Pepsin and carbonic anhydrase isoenzyme III as diagnostic markers for laryngopharyngeal reflux disease. Laryngoscope. 2004;114(12):2129–34.

12. Gill GA, Johnston N, Buda A, et al. Laryngeal epithelial defenses against laryngopharyngeal reflux: investigations of E-cadherin, carbonic anhydrase isoenzyme III, and pepsin. Ann Otol Rhinol Laryngol. 2005;114:913–21.

13. Borges LF, Chan WW, Carroll TL. Dual pH probes without proximal esophageal and pharyngeal impedance may be deficient in diagnosing LPR. J Voice. 2018. pii: S0892-1997(18)30005-5.

14. Liu C, Wang H, Liu K. Meta-analysis of the efficacy of proton pump inhibitors for the symptoms of laryngopharyngeal reflux. Braz J Med Biol Res. 2016;49:e5149.

15. Wei C. A meta-analysis for the role of proton pump inhibitor therapy in patients with laryngopharyngeal reflux. Eur Arch Otorhinolaryngol. 2016;273(11):3795–801.

16. Reichel O, Dressel H, Wiederänders K, Issing WJ. Double-blind, placebo-controlled trial with esomeprazole for symptoms and signs associated with laryngopharyngeal reflux. Otolaryngol Head Neck Surg. 2008;139(3):414–20.

17. Khan M, Santana J, Donnellan C, Preston C, Moayyedi P. Medical treatments in the short term management of reflux oesophagitis. Cochrane Database Syst Rev. 2007;(2):CD003244.

18. Gomm W, von Holt K, Thomé F, Broich K, Maier W, Fink A, Doblhammer G, Haenisch B. Association of proton pump inhibitors with risk of dementia: a pharmacoepidemiological claims data analysis. JAMA Neurol. 2016;73(4):410–6.

19. Batchelor R, Kumar R, Gilmartin-Thomas JFM, Hopper I, Kemp W, Liew D. Systematic review with meta-analysis: risk of adverse cardiovascular events with proton pump inhibitors independent of clopidogrel. Aliment Pharmacol Ther. 2018;48(8):780–96.

20. Van der Hoorn MMC, Tett SE, de Vries OJ, Dobson AJ, Peeters GMEEG. The effect of dose and type of proton pump inhibitor use on risk of fractures and osteoporosis treatment in older Australian women: a prospective cohort study. Bone. 2015;81:675–82.

21. Ngamruengphong S, Leontiadis GI, Radhi S, Dentino A, Nugent K. Proton pump inhibitors and risk of fracture: a systematic review and meta-analysis of observational studies. Am J Gastroenterol. 2011;106(7):1209–18.

22. Nochaiwong S, Ruengorn C, Awiphan R, Koyratkoson K, Chaisai C, Noppakun K, Chongruksut W, Thavorn K. The association between proton pump inhibitor use and the risk of adverse kidney outcomes: a systematic review and meta-analysis. Nephrol Dial Transplant. 2018;33(2):331–42.

23. Imfeld P, Bodmer M, Jick SS, Meier CR. Proton pump inhibitor use and risk of developing Alzheimer's disease or vascular dementia: a case-control analysis. Drug Saf. 2018;41(12):1387–96.

24. Pasternak B, Hviid A. Use of proton-pump inhibitors in early pregnancy and the risk of birth defects. N Engl J Med. 2010;363(22):2114–23.

25. Savarino E, Zentilin P, Marabotto E, Bodini G, Della Coletta M, Frazzoni M, Savarino V. A review of pharmacotherapy for treating gastroesophageal reflux disease (GERD). Expert Opin Pharmacother. 2017;18(13):1333–43.

26. Savarino V, Martinucci I, Furnari M, et al. Vonoprazan for treatment of gastroesophageal reflux: pharmacodynamic and pharmacokinetic considerations. Expert Opin Drug Metab Toxicol. 2016;12(11):1333–41.

27. Vela MF, Camacho-Lobato L, Srinivasan R, et al. Simultaneous intraesophageal impedance and pH measurement of acid and nonacid gastro-

esophageal reflux: effect of omeprazole. Gastroenterology. 2001;120:1599–606.

28. Boeckxstaens GE, Denison H, Jensen JM, et al. Translational gastrointestinal pharmacology in the 21st century: the lesogaberan story. Curr Opin Pharmacol. 2011;11:630–3.

29. Weijenborg PW, de Schepper HS, Smout AJ, et al. Effects of antidepressants in patients with functional esophageal disorders or gastroesophageal reflux disease: a systematic review. Clin Gastroenterol Hepatol. 2015;13:251–9.

30. Blaga Surdea T, Bancilà I, Dobru D, et al. Mucosal protective compounds in the treatment of gastroesophageal reflux disease. A position paper based on evidence of the Romanian Society of Gastroenterology. J Gastrointest Liver Dis. 2016;25:537–46.

31. Reimer C, Lødrup AB, Smith G, et al. Randomised clinical trial: alginate (GavisconAdvance) vs. placebo as add-on therapy in reflux patients with inadequate response to a once daily proton pump inhibitor. Aliment Pharmacol Ther. 2016;43(8):899–909.

32. McGlashan JA, Johnstone LM, Sykes J. The value of a liquid alginate suspension (Gaviscon Advance) in the management of laryngopharyngeal reflux. Eur Arch Otorhinolaryngol. 2009;266(2):243–51.

33. Palmieri B, Corbascio D, Capone S, et al. Preliminary clinical experience with a new natural compound in the treatment of esophagitis and gastritis: symptomatic effect. Trends Med. 2009;9:219–25.

34. Yang J, Dehom S, Sanders S, et al. Treating laryngopharyngeal reflux: evaluation of an anti-reflux program with comparison to medications. Am J Otolaryngol. 2018;39(1):50–5.

35. Zalvan CH, Hu S, Greenberg B, Geliebter J. A comparison of alkaline water and mediterranean diet vs. proton pump inhibition for treatment of laryngopharyngeal reflux. JAMA Otolaryngol Head Neck Surg. 2017;143(10):1023–9.

36. Min C, Park B, Sim S, Choi HG. Dietary modification for laryngopharyngeal reflux: systematic review. J Laryngol Otol. 2019;133(2):80–6.

37. Giacchi RJ, Sullivan D, Rothstein SG. Compliance with anti-reflux therapy in patients with otolaryngologic manifestations of gastroesophageal reflux disease. Laryngoscope. 2000;110(1):19–22.

38. Shaker R, Babaei A, Naini SR. Prevention of esophagopharyngeal reflux by augmenting the upper esophageal sphincter pressure barrier. Laryngoscope. 2014;124(10):2268–74.

39. Yadlapati R, Craft J, Adkins CJ, Pandolfino JE. The upper esophageal sphincter assist device is associated with symptom response in reflux associated laryngeal symptoms. Clin Gastroenterol Hepatol. 2018;16(10):1670–2.

40. Lechien JR, Akst LM, Hamdan AL, et al. Evaluation and management of laryngopharyngeal reflux disease: state of the art review. Otolaryngol Head Neck Surg. 2019;160(5):762–82.

Chronic Cough

7

Christopher D. Dwyer, Juliana K. Litts, and VyVy N. Young

Introduction

With nearly 30 million patient visits in the United States each year, cough ranks among the top five symptoms prompting patients to seek medical advice. By nature of its prevalence, cough is a frequently encountered complaint in tertiary care laryngology clinics. While often transient and attributable to viral respiratory tract illness in the majority of patients, up to 12% of patients report a cough that is chronic in nature [1]. Given the broad differential of etiologies, chronic cough frequently results in extensive investigations, multiple office visits, and numerous specialist referrals including otolaryngology, allergy, pulmonology, and

C. D. Dwyer · V. N. Young (✉)
UCSF Voice and Swallowing Center, Department of Otolaryngology-Head and Neck Surgery, University of California, San Francisco, San Francisco, CA, USA
e-mail: vyvy.young@ucsf.edu

J. K. Litts
Department of Otolaryngology, University of Colorado School of Medicine, Aurora, CO, USA

© Springer Nature Switzerland AG 2021
D. E. Rosow, C. M. Ivey (eds.), *Evidence-Based Laryngology*,
https://doi.org/10.1007/978-3-030-58494-8_7

gastroenterology. The otolaryngologist's role, at the very least, lies in identifying potential upper aerodigestive tract etiologies and optimizing management strategies to improve or alleviate this common complaint.

The most widely accepted classification of cough, established by expert guidelines from the American Academy of Chest Physicians, divides cough into three categories based on symptom duration [2]. An acute cough is present for less than 3 weeks, subacute cough between 3 and 8 weeks, and chronic cough persists for greater than 8 weeks duration. Most cases of acute cough are related to viral respiratory tract illnesses, are usually self-limited in nature, and require no significant treatment or workup. Once a cough becomes chronic, identifying an etiology becomes paramount, and management of the underlying cause is recommended.

Cough Anatomy and Neurophysiology

Understanding a normal physiologic cough response is critical to determining if a patient's cough complaint is physiologic or pathologic. It is a normal protective reflex activity, and preserves the gas exchanging functions of the bronchopulmonary tree [3]. Familiarity with the basic anatomic and neurophysiologic mechanisms generating cough is important for the treating clinician to provide a rational and systematic approach for successful treatment.

Cough is a reflex-mediated modification of the breathing pattern in response to airway irritation. In simplest terms, afferent sensory receptors are activated, the signal is relayed to the medullary cough center, and an efferent motor cough response is generated. Vagal afferent nerves arise from the inferior nodose and superior jugular ganglia and are distributed throughout the bronchopulmonary mucosa [4]. The cough center in the medulla generates an efferent signal that travels down the vagus, phrenic, and spinal motor nerves to expiratory musculature to produce a cough motor response.

Most of what is known about the sensory neuroanatomy of cough has been derived from animal studies, primarily the guinea pig. There are limited in vivo human studies, and thus most of the anatomy and neurophysiology has been inferred [3]. Cough receptors are diffusely distributed throughout the aerodigestive tract, as well as in the pericardium and diaphragm. They are most densely located in the proximal airway, including the larynx, carina, and other airway bifurcations. Given this broad distribution of sensory afferents, the differential diagnosis for cough is vast, overlapping with many different specialties.

Vagal cough afferents are broadly distributed into chemoreceptors and mechanoreceptors. Chemoreceptors are unmyelinated C-fiber nociceptors stimulated by chemical irritants. They express two well-described ion channels: transient receptor vanilloid 1 (TRVP1) and transient receptor ankyrin 1 (TRPA1). These ion channels are selectively activated by capsaicin, bradykinin, and TRPA1 activators [3]. Overexpression of TRPV1 has been demonstrated in chronic cough patients [5]. Capsaicin has also been used in cough desensitization by selectively rendering C-fibers unresponsive to their normal stimuli [6–9]. The other major subset of vagal afferents are myelinated mechanoreceptors. These are stimulated by triggers such as touch or displacement. These are capsaicin insensitive because they do not express TRVP1 or TRPA1 receptors [3, 10, 11].

The central nervous system is known to both modulate and regulate the cough reflex. Convergence of vagal afferents occurs in the brainstem, especially in the nucleus of the solitary tract (nTS). This allows for synergistic regulation of the cough reflex. Central modification of the cough response is thought to play a key role in the enhanced cough responsiveness resulting from allergic inflammation, gastroesophageal reflux disease (GERD), and other upper airway diseases. Here, esophageal and trigeminal afferents may integrate with central cough circuits, resulting in a hyper-responsive cough response [12, 13]. Coughing, like many other functions, is also subject to conscious, higher order control. Both inhibition and voluntary production of cough are possible, and both cough suppression therapy and behavioral modification can be explored as possible strategies to decrease cough behavior.

Chronic Cough Assessment and Workup

History and Physical Examination

The initial approach to a patient with chronic cough is focused on determining likely underlying etiologies and ruling out sinister causes that are potentially life-threatening. A detailed history about the cough should include a sinonasal history, allergens, esophageal and extra-esophageal reflux symptom inquiry, tobacco smoking status (current or previous), and occupational exposures. Red flag symptoms include fever, chills, weight loss, anorexia, night sweats, hemoptysis, cough following oral intake, choking episodes, orthopnea, and chest pain. An urgent workup of these patients is warranted. A comprehensive head and neck examination including complete sinonasal endoscopy and laryngoscopy should also be performed. Videostroboscopy is an adjunct that may reveal less common causes of cough such as glottic insufficiency or subtle vocal fold paresis. Chest auscultation for adventitious lung sounds, rubs, bruits, and murmurs may point toward a lower airway or cardiac cough etiology.

Patients will often report that they have been previously investigated extensively and have trialed medications that were unsuccessful. Unfortunately, patient compliance to empiric treatment trials or duration of the trial are often insufficient to consider them truly negative or unhelpful. Thus, detailed review of previous workups and trialed medications including compliance, duration, and effect on cough symptoms can determine if the trials were indeed adequate.

Medication Review

The most common medication class causing chronic cough is ACE inhibitors. The literature reports an incidence of 2–33% of chronic cough in patients taking an ACE inhibitor [14–17]. Chronic cough can develop at any point during their use, even after years of tolerance, and is not dose-dependent [17]. Cessation of medication and use of an alternative antihypertensive will usually resolve the cough. Resolution of cough typically occurs within 1–4 weeks after the cessation of therapy, but may linger up to 3 months [18]. Angiotensin II receptor antagonists (ARBs) are alternatives to ACE inhibitors that do not affect kinin metabolism. They have not been associated with increased cough incidence, even in patients who have previously had an ACE inhibitor-induced cough [18]. Medications resulting in cough from bronchospasm include B-blockers, NSAIDs, and Aspirin. Bisphosphonates, calcium antagonists, and systemic steroids may cause cough through worsening of gastric reflux. Inhaled corticosteroids (ICS) may paradoxically cause cough as a result of laryngeal irritation or candidiasis.

Diagnostic Testing

The suspected etiology of cough should guide the clinician's choice of additional investigations. At minimum, chest radiography (CXR) is recommended if the patient does not smoke or take an ACE inhibitor, or if the cough persists after withdrawal of medication [19]. Other investigations should be guided by most likely underlying etiologies.

Cough Etiology

The following section briefly outlines the most common causes thought to result in chronic cough. Upper airway cough syndrome (UACS), asthma, and gastroesophageal/laryngopharyngeal reflux disease are cited to represent the three most common causes of chronic cough in adult, nonsmoking patients with normal chest radiography and absence of ACE inhibitor use on medication review. Combined, they represent up to 99.4% of chronic cough cases in prospective series, and cough is multifactorial in up to 59% [20, 21]. They are discussed in more detail below. Table 7.1 provides an overview of other potential chronic cough etiologies to be considered.

Table 7.1 Chronic cough etiologies

Common causes of chronic cough
Tobacco smoking
ACE-inhibitor use
Upper airway cough syndrome
Asthma
Gastroesophageal/laryngopharyngeal reflux disease

Less common causes of chronic cough
Pulmonary
Bronchiectasis
Chronic bronchitis/chronic obstructive pulmonary disease
Non-asthmatic eosinophilic bronchitis
Interstitial lung disease
Lung malignancy
Bronchiolitis
Arteriovenous malformations
Foreign body
Chronic hypersensitivity pneumonitis
Ciliary dyskinesia
Cystic fibrosis
Sarcoidosis
Laryngeal/Hypopharyngeal
Chronic/recurrent aspiration
Hypopharyngeal/Zenker's diverticulum
Cricopharyngeal web/bar
Paradoxical vocal fold motion disorder
Glottic insufficiency (atrophy, vocal fold paralysis, sulcus vocalis, vocal fold paresis)
Laryngeal malignancy
Infectious/Post-infectious
Post-infectious cough
Pertussis
Lung abscess
Tuberculosis
Mediastinal
Congestive heart failure
Pericarditis
Retrosternal goiter
Fibrosing mediastinitis
Acute pulmonary embolism
Other
Cerumen impaction
External auditory canal irritation
Habitual cough
Somatization disorder
Multiple chemical sensitivity

Upper Airway Cough Syndrome

In 2006, the American Academy of Chest Physicians published an updated set of cough guidelines. They proposed the terminology "upper airway cough syndrome" in place of postnasal drip syndrome. UACS is a nonspecific term that encompasses a variety of sinonasal diseases resulting in cough as a presenting symptom. This entity is considered the most common etiology of chronic cough [22]. The most commonly encountered upper airway conditions resulting in chronic cough include allergic rhinitis, chronic rhinosinusitis, and nonallergic rhinitis (NAR). A brief overview of these selected sinonasal diseases is reviewed, and evidence-based treatment modalities are provided.

A strong body of evidence supports consideration of the upper and lower airways as a single functional unit. This has been described as the *unified airway* model. Worsening of disease and inflammation in one area of the airway is known to result in a negative impact on the other. Similarly, effective treatment management in one area often results in improvement within other airway sites. For this reason, the otolaryngologist should thoroughly investigate the nasal airway and paranasal sinuses, and address these areas as potential etiologies for chronic cough. The unified airway model has been proposed to extend to both the middle ear cleft and possibly the larynx as well [23].

Chronic rhinosinusitis is defined by the presence of subjective clinical symptoms (e.g. nasal congestion, obstruction, mucopurulent drainage, facial pain-pressure-fullness, and altered sense of smell) and objective evidence of sinonasal inflammation (i.e. endoscopic purulence/edema, polyposis, or radiographic evidence of paranasal sinus inflammation). In chronic rhinosinusitis with nasal polyposis (CRSwNP), the prevalence of asthma is up to 50% [24]. Medical and surgical management has been proven to improve both asthma control and asthma-specific medication usage [24].

Allergic rhinitis is an inflammatory, IgE-mediated disease process that presents as nasal congestion and obstruction, rhinorrhea, sneezing, and pruritus. Physical exam findings of sinonasal inflammation include turbinate hypertrophy, nasal secretions, or middle meatal and nasal mucosal edema. Allergy testing will commonly identify a positive response to specific allergy antigens on skin prick testing. A positive treatment response to both sinonasal and cough symptoms is strongly suggestive of AR as the cause of UACS. Nonallergic rhinitis is classified by similar nasal symptoms, but no allergic antigens are identified, and the disease process is non-IgE mediated. NAR is classified into inflammatory and noninflammatory etiologies, and both can result in cough as an included symptom.

Medical management strategies for the above conditions are similar, and thus may be trialed before extensive testing and investigations are offered. A positive response to medical management with cough improvement supports a diagnosis of upper airway cough syndrome, and may alleviate the need for expensive testing. An empiric trial of medications supported by evidence-based medicine includes first-generation antihistamines (e.g. diphenhydramine, hydroxyzine, and chlorpheniramine) and an inhaled nasal corticosteroid spray (e.g. beclomethasone, budesonide, ciclesonide, fluticasone, or mometasone) [25, 26]. Pratter and colleagues showed that 59% of patients responded to first-generation-decongestant therapy alone, and an additional 33% responded to first-generation decongestant with nasal corticosteroid [27]. Most studies on cough suppression use first-generation antihistamines because of their anticholinergic activity [28]. Thus, although both first- and second-generation antihistamines are competitive antagonists to histamine at the H1-receptor site, evidence is currently limited to first-generation medications for the treatment of cough in UACS. Second-generation antihistamines (e.g. loratidine, fexofenadine, terfenadine, or cetirizine) have not been shown to affect the cough reflex [28–30].

Nasal steroid sprays are the most effective long-term treatment options for controlling nasal symptoms associated with allergic rhinitis. Mometasone nasal spray has proven efficacy in relieving daytime cough as well as nasal symptoms of seasonal allergic rhinitis [25, 26, 31]. An empiric trial of inhaled nasal sprays may provide symptomatic benefit for chronic cough in the case of postviral or otherwise asymptomatic patients. A small prospective trial by Macedo et al. evaluated treatment outcomes with fluticasone, ipratropium, and azelastine nasal sprays on patients with chronic cough and the sensation of postnasal drip. In 18 patients who completed the study, 28% reported an overall improvement in their cough scores following treatment. However, there was no improvement in Leicester Cough Questionnaire (LCQ) scores or capsaicin cough responses. Improved anterior nasal discharge and endoscopic nasal scores, however, were other notable findings. They concluded a potential modest improvement in cough could be achieved with triple modality nasal therapy [32].

Randomized control trials (RCT) assessing the efficacy of inhaled anticholinergics are largely lacking, and reported studies provide contradictory results. Inhaled agents such as tiotropium, ipratropium, and oxitropium in patients with post-viral cough syndrome or acute URI have not been conclusive [30, 33, 34]. It is uncertain if these findings also apply to chronic cough patients with concurrent upper respiratory tract disease.

Nasal irrigations with saline have proven beneficial in alleviating nasal symptoms and quality of life (QOL) [35–37]. This basic nasal hygiene intervention is promoted in the management of most inflammatory nasal diseases including AR, NAR, and CRS. High-volume irrigation of the nose and paranasal sinuses aid in the removal of debris, mucus and crusting, allergens, and irritants, with potential improvement in both nasal symptoms and cough [38].

Numerous other agents have been tried for treatment of upper airway inflammatory disease. These studies, however, assess efficacy on sinonasal symptoms, and not specifically cough itself. These include xylitol, Manuka honey, colloidal silver, and other surfactants [39–42]. These agents require further investigation, specifically with regard to their effects on cough, before evidence-based recommendations can be made.

Level of evidence	Conclusion
3	Fluticasone, ipratropium, and azelastine nasal sprays may make modest improvement in cough symptoms [32]

Asthma

Asthma is thought to represent the second leading cause of chronic cough in nonsmoking adults. Symptoms of wheeze, shortness of breath, chest tightness, and cough are the cardinal presenting symptoms. In a subset of patients, however, cough is the predominant and sometimes only symptom, thus giving rise to the term cough variant asthma. The key feature of all asthma variants is variable expiratory airflow restriction. The diagnosis is based on an appropriate history, exclusion of other diagnoses, and the demonstration of variable airflow obstruction using spirometry. The forced expiratory volume in 1 second (FEV1) is compared to forced vital capacity (FVC). A FEV1/FVC ratio less than 0.7 is the threshold for defining airway obstruction via spirometry. Variability in airflow obstruction can be demonstrated using bronchodilator reversibility. An increased FEV1 of 12% and absolute change of 200 cc is used to define a positive response. Alternatively, bronchoprovocation testing with methacholine can be used to induce bronchoconstriction [43].

Asthma management typically consists of anti-inflammatory modulators such as inhaled or systemic corticosteroids, short- or long-acting inhaled bronchodilator B-agonists, leukotriene inhibitors, methylxanthines (i.e. theophylline), and mast cell stabilizers (i.e. cromolyn and nedrocromil). Anti-IgE monoclonal antibodies (e.g. omalizumab) are also effective but usually reserved for severe, refractory cases.

Non-asthmatic eosinophilic bronchitis is another condition of which the otolaryngologist should be aware. The reported frequency of this entity as a cause of chronic cough varies in different reports but has been suggested to represent between 10% and 15% of cases presenting to a specialist clinic [44]. This condition presents with eosinophilic inflammation of the airway epithelium without evidence of bronchoconstriction. The diagnosis is confirmed by an induced sputum demonstrating eosinophilia or via fractional exhaled nitric oxide testing, and the condition is usually responsive to inhaled corticosteroids [45].

Gastric Reflux Disease

The pathophysiologic mechanism by which gastric reflux causes chronic cough is debated and incompletely understood. Nonetheless, there is a clinically evident association between refluxate of gastric contents into the esophagus and laryngopharynx and chronic cough. Cough is a commonly listed symptom among the extra esophageal symptoms in GERD questionnaires. Both acid and nonacid reflux are potentially causative.

Similar to cough variant asthma, patients with cough who lack other classic reflux symptoms may nonetheless demonstrate evidence of gastric reflux using investigations such as impedance-pH monitoring. This condition, referred to as "silent reflux," may be accountable for up to 75% of reflux-induced chronic cough [46]. Unfortunately, as discussed later in this chapter, treatment directed toward acid suppression does not always alleviate the symptom of cough itself.

One challenge encountered when reviewing the available literature for improvement in cough with reflux therapy is the variability in reflux symptoms (e.g. heartburn, regurgitation) and/or objective measures (i.e. endoscopy, 24-hr pH testing, or impedance testing) used as inclusion and exclusion criteria. Hence, there exists considerable heterogeneity within the published study populations. Even more controversial is the inconsistency in the diagnosis of laryngopharyngeal reflux disease and its implications on chronic cough.

Available prospective studies have generated conflicting and equivocal results on the efficacy of proton pump inhibitors for treatment of suspected reflux-related cough. Two small randomized control trials concluded that proton-pump inhibitor (PPI) therapy with omeprazole may improve cough symptoms. These studies utilized 24-hr pH testing as confirmation of acid reflux disease, thus excluding patients with nonacid or weakly acidic reflux [47, 48].

A Cochrane analysis found insufficient evidence that PPIs are universally beneficial for GERD-related cough [49]. Another systematic review of 11 studies with meta-analysis of five of these studies was published in 2006. Outcome measures for all the studies were various subjective cough scales, and none used objective monitoring of cough. Several brands and doses of PPIs were used, and criteria for suspected GERD-related cough were variable. They found favorable outcomes for PPIs, and concluded that PPIs for cough associated with GERD probably have some effect in some adults, though the effect is less universal than reported in cohort studies. This publication concurrently recommended that additional RCTs be designed using valid cough outcomes to justify international guidelines that currently recommend an empirical trial of PPIs for suspected reflux-related cough [50, 51].

In 2016, the *CHEST* journal published an updated set of recommendations and guidelines regarding cough-reflux syndrome based on a review of the literature by an expert cough panel. The recommendations from this publication are based on a review of 14 randomized control trials assessing outcomes following treatment of suspected reflux-related cough. The expert panel concluded that if patients report heartburn and regurgitation in addition to their cough, that a trial of PPIs, H2-receptor antagonists, alginate, or antacids is reasonable. Studies that included lifestyle modifications and weight loss had better cough outcomes. Finally, in the absence of heartburn or indigestion, it was discouraged to use PPI therapy alone as this has not been effective in consistently resolving cough. A well-detailed summary of these RCTs is provided in the 2016 *CHEST* publication [52].

Level of evidence	Conclusion
1	In adult patients with suspected chronic cough due to reflux-cough syndrome, and typical symptoms of reflux and regurgitation, a PPI trial in addition to lifestyle modification and weight loss may improve cough
	In the absence of heartburn or regurgitation, use of PPIs in isolation have not consistently been shown to resolve cough [52]

Positive outcomes using laparoscopic fundoplication have been reported in the literature for improving cough associated with reflux disease. Kaufman and colleagues retrospectively reported their long-term outcomes of 128 patients treated with laparoscopic anti-reflux surgery. Cough was reported preoperatively in 85% of patients ($n = 108$), and postoperatively improved in 74% (80/108) and resolved in 41% (44/108) [53]. Another retrospective study of 54 patients with evidence of reflux and cough underwent laparoscopic Nissan fundoplication. Follow-up at 3 months resulted in 70.4% of patients being free of cough, 22.2% with significant improvement in cough, and 7.4% who were unchanged. Cough in appropriately selected patients disappeared for the majority of their cohort shortly following laparoscopic anti-reflux surgery, and consideration of surgery was recommended for this patient complaint [54]. In a meta-analysis of 25 studies, improvement in extra-esophageal symptoms (including, but not limited to, cough) was variable, with 15–95% reporting improvement following surgical fundoplication [55]. These studies are limited again by nonrandomization and variable selection criteria. Additional prospective and randomized studies are needed to investigate the effectiveness of surgical reflux management on chronic cough.

Level of evidence	Conclusion
3	Improvement in chronic cough following laparoscopic anti-reflux surgery has been demonstrated in numerous retrospective series, but with variable success rates [55]

Chronic Cough Terminology

Unfortunately, despite thorough history, investigations, and empiric trials of medications directed toward the most common causes of chronic cough, some patients remain symptomatic and affected by their cough. Persistent cough of unexplained origin occurs in up to 10% of patients seeking assistance for chronic cough [19], and upwards of 46% of patients referred to a specialty cough clinic [56].

The term unexplained chronic cough is utilized in the 2016 *CHEST* guidelines. This term encompasses patients with cough of greater than 8 weeks duration that is persistent despite appropriate investigation and treatment. This publication also makes note of explained but refractory cough when a patient is identified to have conditions associated with chronic cough, but the cough persists after treatment of these etiologies. An unexplained refractory cough is a term reserved for patients with negative investigations who do not respond to empiric therapy trials [57].

A review of the literature gives rise to a variety of different terms to describe cough that is of unknown etiology or refractory to management. These include unexplained chronic cough, refractory chronic cough, idiopathic chronic cough, chronic cough of unknown etiology, chronic treatment-resistant cough, intractable chronic cough, neurogenic cough, cough hypersensitivity syndrome, and post-viral vagal neuropathy. Unfortunately, most of these terms do not have rigorous definitions, and are not consistently applied. The reader should keep this in mind when reviewing the literature and the evidence-based summaries provided in this chapter.

One "category" of terminology used to describe chronic cough warrants further discussion, given its relevance to the otolaryngologist. Neurogenic cough is a term that has been proposed as an etiology for chronic cough likely related to neuropathy or nerve dysfunction [58]. This type of cough has also often been reserved as a diagnosis of exclusion. The term laryngeal hypersensitivity syndrome, sometimes referred to as cough hypersensitivity syndrome, on the other hand, encompasses a broad number of vague laryngeal symptoms in addition to cough, such as globus, throat clearing, throat tickle/irritation, and dysphonia [59]. The term irritable larynx syndrome was first coined by Morrison and colleagues in 1999 [60]. They described a hyperfunctional, spasm-ready laryngeal state easily triggered by sensory stimuli such as odors, foods, voice use, or refluxate. The development of this condition was proceeded by a viral illness in 17/39 cases. Other authors have described a similar chronic cough condition, described as post-viral vagal neuropathy (PVVN), associated with abnormal laryngeal EMG findings of neuropathy [61]. In addition to these commonly used terms is laryngeal sensory neuropathy [62]. This term has been used to denote chronic cough in association with evidence of vagal neuropathy, not necessarily as a result of viral illness. The multitude of different terms for relatively similar cough variants can be confusing, and leads to interchangeable use of different terms likely describing a cough process with similar underlying pathophysiology.

Pharmacological Management Options for Cough

The following section outlines pharmacologic treatments that have been trialed for chronic cough. These are of particular utility for unexplained chronic cough and cough of suspected neurogenic origin. The best quality evidence for these treatment considerations is provided.

Neuromodulators

Neuromodulating medications have proven efficacy in the treatment of chronic cough, supported by numerous high quality randomized control trials. These medications have been shown to improve both cough severity and cough related QOL [63–65]. The most commonly employed agents include gabapentin, pregabalin, amitriptyline, baclofen, and tramadol. There is level 1 evidence supporting the use of gabapentin, pregabalin, and amitriptyline as discussed below. These medications traditionally have been used in the treatment of neurogenic cough and laryngeal hypersensitivity syndromes.

It is thought that potentiation of the normal cough reflex in neurogenic cough is the result of three potential mechanisms. One includes a lowered threshold for stimulation of sensory afferents [59]. Additionally, spontaneous activation of receptors has been proposed as an explanation of the commonly reported symptom of "throat tickle" that precedes the cough in many patients [66]. Finally, central modulation of the cough reflex is another potential etiology. This central sensitization results in an amplification of afferent inputs arriving at the solitary nucleus with resultant cough [58, 59].

A randomized control trial by Jeyakumar et al. demonstrated significant improvement in cough severity and QOL with a 10 day course of amitriptyline. Amitriptyline is a tricyclic antidepressant that predominantly inhibits the re-uptake of serotonin and norepinephrine. The advantages of this medication include numerous prospective studies supporting its use [63, 65–67] and once daily dosing titration regime. Caution should be exercised in the elderly due to its anticholinergic side effects. A potential alternative in patients older than 65 years is nortriptyline, which reportedly has less side effects than its counterpart [68]. The efficacy of this medication, however, is not yet supported by prospective or retrospective evidence-based medicine. Typical dosing of amitriptyline in prospective studies includes initiating medication at 10 mg daily, and titrating upwards to 100 mg as tolerated and until cough symptoms are adequately controlled.

Both gabapentin and pregabalin are gamma aminobutyric acid (GABA) analogs, and they inhibit voltage-gated calcium channel neurotransmitter release. Both agents have level 1 randomized control trial evidence supporting their efficacy in the treatment of chronic cough. Ryan et al. in 2012 published in *Lancet* on the efficacy of gabapentin in a double-blind RCT. Unfortunately, the effect on cough severity was lost within 4 weeks of discontinuing medication [65]. Usual dosing is 100 mg three times daily, titrated upwards to 1800 mg (600 mg TID).

Pregabalin has demonstrated efficacy in prospective studies and RCTs as well. An RCT by Vertigan et al. employed a pregabalin titration regime in addition to four sessions of speech therapy. The placebo arm included four sessions of speech therapy only. Similar to gabapentin, however, upon discontinuation of medication, at 18 weeks the treatment effect was lost with respect to cough severity and cough-related quality of life [64]. Pregabalin is usually started at a dose of 75 mg daily and titrated upwards to 300 mg total daily.

Baclofen and tramadol are other potential neuromodulating agents that can be considered for chronic cough management. These agents are typically used as second line options after failing one of the aforementioned agents or when side effects are not tolerated [68]. A prospective cohort study by Dion et al. in 2017 showed efficacy of tramadol in the treatment of neurogenic cough [69]. In this series, 16 patients with neurogenic cough were given tramadol 50 mg every 8 hours as needed, and subjects were included if patients completed the Cough Severity Index (CSI) and LCQ before and after 14 days of treatment. Concerns are often raised about this medication; however, due to its weak opioid agonist activity and potential for dependence [70]. Baclofen, which has GABA agonist properties, has been shown to increase the cough threshold response to irritants such as capsaicin [71]. Its use in chronic cough is limited to a two-person crossover case report. Both patients had decreased cough severity when baclofen was prescribed at a dose of 10 mg TID × 14 days [72].

Mechanisms by which neuromodulating medications alleviate symptoms of chronic cough remain unknown. Most RCTs demonstrate benefit of these medications; however, effect is generally lost following discontinuation of medication in the aforementioned published studies. Thus, the potential for long-term efficacy, duration of treatment, and optimal dosing remain to be determined. A systematic review published by Cohen and Misono in 2013 failed to demonstrate any definite superior agent, length of therapy, or follow-up course [73]. Eight relevant articles were reviewed including two RCTs and two prospective studies. A broad range of neuromodulators were assessed including pregabalin, gabapentin, amitriptyline, and baclofen. Improvements in cough-specific quality of life and severity resulted from neuromodulator therapy, and further studies with design improvements would likely contribute to better understanding of the efficacy, optimal treatment duration and dosing of these agents. A best practice article was also recently published in Laryngoscope in 2017 regarding the efficacy of neuromodulating agents for cough. Based on best available reviewed literature, the use of neuromodulators appears to be helpful in patients with chronic idiopathic/neurogenic cough [74].

Level of evidence	Conclusion
1	Neuromodulators such as gabapentin, amitriptyline, and pregabalin have demonstrated efficacy in the treatment of chronic cough, but treatment effect is generally lost following discontinuation [63–65]

Inhaled Corticosteroids

The role of inhaled corticosteroids in the management of a patient with chronic cough is largely focused on the treatment of asthma and pulmonary disease. While the efficacy of ICSs is well established for the treatment of asthma and its variants, their role in the treatment of chronic cough not attributable to asthma and its variants remains controversial. The most recent

2016 *CHEST* guidelines suggested that inhaled corticosteroids should not be prescribed for adult patients with unexplained chronic cough and negative testing for bronchial hyperresponsiveness and eosinophilia (i.e. sputum eosinophils, exhaled nitric oxide) [57]. At least three high-quality RCTs have investigated the role of inhaled corticosteroids in unexplained chronic cough. Their conclusions regarding effectiveness of ICSs show conflicting results.

Pizzichini et al. conducted a randomized, double-blind study enrolling 44 adult non-asthmatic, negative sputum eosinophilia patients to either placebo or budesonide 400 mg twice daily for 2 weeks. They excluded chronic cough patients with bronchial hyperresponsiveness and positive induced sputum testing for eosinophils. They found no beneficial effect of inhaled budesonide in this study cohort. No effect on cough discomfort as measured by visual analog scale was noted on follow-up [75].

The other two high-quality studies included in the recent *CHEST* guidelines unfortunately did not perform bronchial hypersensitivity or induced sputum testing as part of their enrollment testing. Thus, a portion of their unexplained chronic cough patients may have actually had asthma or eosinophilic bronchitis. Ribeiro et al. assessed inhaled beclomethasone in a prospective, randomized, double-blind, placebo-controlled study enrolling 64 patients [76]. Of note, half the patients included in this study had positive bronchial hypersensitivity testing results in follow-up, and therefore would have been expected to improve with ICSs. There was, however, a subset of 15 patients with negative bronchopulmonary testing that responded to treatment. Unfortunately, induced sputum to assess for eosinophilic bronchitis was not performed and this cause of chronic cough could not be excluded [76]. Finally, Chaudhuri and colleagues demonstrated a partial response to inhaled fluticasone as well as reduction in induced sputum concentrations of eosinophilic cationic proteins in a double-blind, randomized, placebo controlled crossover study [77].

Level of evidence	Conclusion
1	Randomized control trials assessing the efficacy of ICSs for the treatment of unexplained chronic cough show mixed results [75–77]

Johnstone et al. published a systematic review reporting on the role of inhaled corticosteroids for unexplained chronic cough. Eight eligible RCTs were included with a total of 570 patients. The studies demonstrated significant heterogeneity, and some RCTs did not exclude patients with upper airway cough syndrome and reflux as potential chronic cough etiologies. Overall, ICS treatment was associated with a decrease in cough score, but the primary outcome of cough cure could not be determined as heterogeneity precluded meta-analysis [78].

Proton Pump Inhibitors

Esomeprazole 20 mg twice daily was compared to placebo in a prospective, single center, double blind, randomized controlled parallel study of 8 weeks duration [79]. The included patients supposedly had clinical features suggestive of reflux-related cough; however, the only two features detailed were cough with phonation and bending in association with food. Heartburn and dyspepsia were not required, no diagnostic reflux testing was performed, and other common etiologies were supposedly excluded. Primary outcome was change in integral response score for cough severity and frequency graded from 0 (best) to 9 (worst). Secondary outcomes included cough symptomatology measured using the LCQ and Hull Airway Reflux Questionnaire. Fifty patients were randomized equally to both the treatment and placebo arms. No differences between the groups were found for any of the measured endpoints; however, improvement in both arms was noted compared to baseline. The authors conclude esomeprazole did not have a clinically important effect greater than placebo for cough, and that a placebo effect may be responsible for symptom improvement [79].

Another study assessed the efficacy of high-dose esomeprazole (40 mg twice daily for 12 weeks) on unexplained chronic cough [80]. An important difference in this study was that patients were not suspected to have reflux-related cough, and other common etiologies were previously addressed and eliminated as suspected causes of cough. The patients reported rare heartburn and had negative studies including 24-hr pH/impedance study, methacholine challenge test, and laryngoscopy. Forty subjects were enrolled and randomized. No benefits on cough severity or quality of life were observed. Based on this study, the 2016 *CHEST* guidelines recommended that in adult patients with unexplained chronic cough and a negative workup for acid reflux disease, proton pump inhibitor therapy should not be prescribed [57]. No recommendations were made, however, about the utility of a trial of PPI/acid suppression in patients with chronic cough without typical reflux symptoms.

Level of evidence	Conclusion
1	In patients with negative reflux testing and without reflux-related symptoms, esomeprazole had no significant effect on cough severity or QOL [79]

Antibiotics

Long-term, low-dose macrolides have been used successfully to treat respiratory conditions such as asthma associated with neutrophilic inflammation of the airways, with subsequent reduction in sputum neutrophil counts [81–83]. Patients with chronic cough have also been shown to have elevated induced sputum neutrophilia and raised concentrations of mediators associated with neutrophilic airway inflammation such as IL-8, TNF-alpha, and PGE2 [84]. These data support a hypothesis that macrolide antibiotics which have anti-neutrophil effects independent of their antimicrobial efficacy might be useful in the treatment of chronic cough. Trials with azithromycin and erythromycin, however, have not demonstrated clinical benefit.

A randomized trial enrolling 30 patients with unexplained chronic cough found no reduction in 24 hour cough frequency or severity when treated with erythromycin 250 mg vs. placebo for 12 weeks in a double-blind, parallel group study. Interestingly, there was a reduction in induced sputum neutrophil count, but this did not translate into clinical cough improvement [85].

Similarly, the use of azithromycin was examined in a randomized, controlled trial that assigned 44 patients with treatment-resistant cough to azithromycin 250 mg or placebo three times weekly for 8 weeks duration. There was no significant improvement in LCQ score compared with placebo. Looking at subgroups of responders, there was a large and significant improvement in LCQ in patients with chronic cough and a concurrent diagnosis of asthma who received azithromycin [86]. The study was not designed to detect subgroup effects and therefore this finding warrants further investigation.

Level of evidence	Conclusion
1	Long-term, low-dose macrolide antibiotics have not demonstrated benefit in improving cough severity or frequency in patients with unexplained or treatment-resistant chronic cough [85, 86]

Oral Corticosteroids

The efficacy of oral corticosteroids for the treatment of chronic cough is extremely limited. A well-powered study conducted for subacute (3–4 weeks duration) post-viral cough demonstrated no significant difference in duration of moderately bad or worse cough nor severity of symptoms compared to the placebo arm [87]. This was a multicenter, placebo-controlled randomized trial investigating the efficacy of oral prednisolone 40 mg daily × 5 days for cough following acute respiratory tract illness. A total of 398 patients completed the study, and primary outcome measures included duration of cough and mean severity score of six common viral respiratory illness symptoms, one of which was cough [87]. However, it is unknown if this conclusion can be extended to cough lasting greater than 8 weeks.

A single double-blind RCT investigating oral prednisolone was identified comparing honey+caffeine, oral corticosteroid, and guaifenesin [88]. The recruited cohort included 97 patients with persistent post-infectious cough of greater than 3 weeks duration, and excluded those with other identifiable etiologies of chronic cough. The mean duration of cough was 2.9 (standard deviation 2.4) months; therefore, some of these patients indeed met criteria for chronic cough. Changes in cough frequency was significant ($p < 0.05$) in both the honey+caffeine (20.8 g honey and 2.9 g of coffee TID) and oral prednisolone (13.3 mg TID) groups, but not the guaifenesin group. However, the method of assessing cough frequency was not evaluated using standardized cough questionnaires or assessment tools, and ultimately a physician categorized the cough on a 4 point Likert-type scale (0–3). The oral prednisolone group mean frequency of cough changed from 3.0 to 2.4, which is still of moderate severity. Of note, honey+caffeine was found to be superior to systemic steroid in the treatment of post-infectious chronic cough [88].

Dextromethorphan and Opiates

Opiates are thought to suppress cough by centrally mediated effects on the cough center, and have been long used as a treatment method to suppress cough. Despite widespread use, studies demonstrating efficacy are limited. Major reservations with using opiates for chronic cough management include side effects (i.e. constipation and somnolence) and risk for dependency.

Codeine has traditionally been one of the most commonly prescribed opiates for antitussive effects. A systematic review suggested that codeine was more effective than placebo in reducing cough severity and frequency. The quality of available studies however was judged to be fair or poor; thus, the conclusions should be viewed with caution [89]. In a randomized trial, 64 subjects with subacute cough were randomly assigned to one of three treatment arms. These included codeine (30 mg twice daily), an investigational nociceptive opioid receptor 1 (NOP1) agonist (SCH486757), or placebo. Cough counts with codeine were reduced relative to placebo, but the effect was not statistically significant [90]. Typical dosing of codeine ranges between 30 and 60 mg every 4–6 hours as needed.

Morphine has level 1 evidence supporting its use in chronic refractory cough. A randomized, double-blind, placebo-controlled trial using 4 weeks of slow release morphine sulphate recruited 27 patients. Dose escalation up to 10 mg twice daily was used. A 40% reduction in cough scores was noted among patients randomized to morphine sulfate. Response to treatment occurred within 5 days and was sustained throughout the 4 weeks of the study period [91]. Of note, despite randomized control trial evidence for its efficacy, the *CHEST* expert cough panel did not pass a recommendation for the use of morphine in chronic unexplained cough [57].

Level of evidence	Conclusion
1/2	Slow-release morphine sulphate at doses of 5–10 mg twice daily decreases cough symptoms and cough reflex sensitivity [91]

Dextromethorphan is a non-opioid agent commonly used for cough. It is available over the counter and included in many combination cough and cold medications. In a systematic review, six studies were identified that compared dextromethorphan versus placebo in the treatment of chronic cough. Overall, dextromethorphan was found to decrease cough severity and frequency modestly in all but one of these studies [89]. This systematic review also identified studies that have compared codeine and dextro-methorphan. The results were variable with only a limited number of subjects in each study [89]. In a cross-over study of 16 patients with chronic cough, codeine and dextromethorphan were equally effective in reducing cough frequency, but dextromethorphan was more effective in reducing cough intensity [92]. It was also the preferred reported anti-tussive by the majority of patients.

Oral Capsaicin

Capsaicin, 8-methyl-N-vanillyl-6-nonenamide, is a chemical derived from chili fruits. This chemical has been used to induce coughing in a controlled, dose dependent, and safe manner [93]. It is an agonist of the respiratory tract sensory C-fibers via TRPV1, as discussed in the pathophysiology section of this chapter. In many chronic cough patients, capsaicin sensitivity is increased, and this is thought to be linked to cough hypersensi-tivity [94–96].

Ternesten-Hasseus and colleagues sought to determine if oral intake of natural capsaicin could desensitize the cough reflex and improve unexplained chronic cough [97]. Twenty four patients with irritant-induced unexplained chronic cough of at least 1 year duration and a positive capsaicin sensitivity test were enrolled, along with 15 controls without a history of cough or respiratory disease. This was a double-blind, crossover, randomized trial. The active treatment protocol consisted of 4 weeks of oral capsaicin (0.4 mg twice daily × 2 weeks, followed by 0.8 mg twice daily × 2 weeks). Regular oral intake of pure capsaicin from chili fruits decreased capsaicin cough sensitivity and improved cough symp-toms and scores as measured by a symptom diary on a scale of 0–3 and the Hull cough questionnaire. Complete resolution of cough was not reported in this study; however, their results sug-gest that patients still reported cough during the last week of active treatment (77.3% mild/moderate, 13.6% severe). Important limitations addressed in the publication include inadequate power, and use of a reflux cough questionnaire rather than a validated questionnaire such as LCQ. As such, conclusions should be inter-preted with caution.

Level of evidence	Conclusion
1/2	Capsaicin powder taken orally reduces cough reflex sensitivity and cough symptoms, but not cough frequency [97]

Inhaled Anticholinergics

Research has identified an inhibitory effect of inhaled anticholinergics on TRPV1 receptors, as well as an attenuation of capsaicin-evoked cough [98, 99]. They may potentially block the efferent limb of the cough reflex and decrease stimulation of cough receptors by alteration of mucociliary factors. Chronic cough following viral respiratory tract illness is also associated with bronchial hyperactivity and positive methacholine challenge [19]. Upregulation of the expression of cough receptors has been proposed, but no definite pathophysiology has yet been elicited [100]. Inhaled anticholinergics such as ipratropium and tiotropium may therefore have a role in the management of patients with chronic cough.

High-quality studies evaluating the efficacy of inhaled anticholinergics are lacking. A small and dated randomized control trial examined the clinical effects of ipratropium bromide in a cross-over study of 14 patients [33]. This study cohort had persistent cough refractory to other treatments and no evidence of asthma or upper airway cough syndrome. Inhaled ipratropium bromide (4 × 20 mcg puffs four times daily, 320 mcg/day) resulted in less daytime and nighttime cough in 12 patients, and complete resolution of cough in 5 patients. The efficacy of ipratropium has been demonstrated in an additional RCT looking at subacute post-infectious viral cough [100], but its effectiveness has not been replicated in chronic cough patients.

Novel Agents

P2X3 receptors are ATP-gated ion channels selectively located on populations of primary afferent nerves arising from both cranial and dorsal root ganglia. These receptors are thought to be expressed in vagal C-fibers innervating the airways based on animal studies [101, 102]. It is thought that P2X3-receptor activation could enhance responsiveness to a broad range of stimuli, as seen in chronic cough patients who demonstrate increased sensitivity to inhaled tussive agents such as capsaicin, citric acid, hypertonic saline, and mannitol. In a proof of concept, randomized, cross-over trial of 24 subjects with refractory cough greater than 8 weeks duration, an investigational P2X3 antagonist (AF-219) decreased mean daytime cough frequency during the two-week study blocks by 75% compared with placebo [103]. Refractory cough included patients in whom no identifiable etiology was elicited or those who were refractory to targeted treatment efforts. However, taste disturbance was noted in all patients taking AF-219 and caused six subjects to withdraw from the study; nausea was also common (38%). These results support a role for P2X3 receptor hypersensitivity in refractory cough, but further study is needed to determine safety and efficacy in a larger number of patients, potentially using a lower dose.

Inhalation of capsaicin evokes coughing through activation of the TRPV1 receptors present on airway afferent C-fibers. This is an attractive potential target in the treatment of chronic cough. SB-705498 is a highly selective and potent antagonist of the human TRPV1 receptor. A double-blind, randomized, placebo-controlled crossover trial with SB-705498 enrolled 21 patients with refractory chronic cough presenting to a specialist cough clinic. Despite a significant reduction in induced cough responses to capsaicin with SB-705498 compared to placebo at 2 hours post treatment, this did not translate into clinically significant improvement in cough at 2 weeks. This study failed to demonstrate any significant durable improvement in patient reported cough severity, urge to cough or cough- specific quality of life compared to placebo [104].

Similarly, another TRPV1 antagonist (XEN-D0501) substantially reduced maximal cough response to capsaicin but did not affect spontaneous awake cough frequency. These results mirror those of SB-705498. This was also a double-blind, randomized, placebo crossover trial enrolling 20 patients with refractory chronic cough to evaluate the antitussive efficacy of 14-day treatment with XEN-D0501 (oral 4 mg twice daily) compared to placebo with a 14-day washout period before the crossover treatment period [105]. These two studies challenge the assumption that changes in capsaicin thresholds imply clinical changes in anti-tussive effects.

Level of evidence	Conclusion
1/2	TRPV1 agents demonstrate reduced cough responses to inhaled capsaicin, but no clinically significant improved cough frequency has been demonstrated in randomized clinical trials [104]
1	P2X3 receptor antagonist AF-219 has a potential anti-tussive effect in patients with refractory chronic cough based on a single, phase 2 randomized, placebo controlled trial [103]

Procedural Management of Chronic Cough

Superior Laryngeal Nerve Block

The use of superior laryngeal nerve (SLN) block for chronic cough is limited to two retrospective case series and has been described only for the treatment of suspected neurogenic cough [106, 107]. In both studies, neurogenic cough was diagnosed upon exclusion and negative workup of other causes of chronic cough and after review of potential cough-inducing medications. SLN block is hypothesized to alter the sensory feedback via the SLN and therefore disrupt the afferent cough signaling pathway [106].

Simpson et al. first published a retrospective study on the use of SLN block for neurogenic cough in 2018. His protocol for treatment included 2 mL of a 50:50 solution of long acting corticosteroid (either triamcinolone amcinolone acetonide 200 mg/5 mL or methylprednisolone 80 mg/1 mL) and a local anesthetic (1% lidocaine with 1:100,000 epinephrine or 0.5% bupivacaine) injected at the entry point of the SLN into the thyrohyoid membrane. They noted that palpation of this area frequently acted as a trigger point for eliciting a cough or patient-reported discomfort. Among their patients, 83.3% (n = 15/18) noted improvement in their self-reported CSI (26.8–14.6), with a mean of 2.4 injections at a mean interval of 41.5 days [106].

A subsequent retrospective case series of ten patients was published in 2019 with a similar injection technique and inclusion criteria. This case series excluded patients previously or concurrently treated with neuromodulating agents. A success rate of 100% improvement in the CSI was reported, with a mean improvement of 6.30 (CI 11.44–21.16, p < 0.001) [107].

Level of evidence	Conclusion
4	The use of superior laryngeal nerve block for treatment of neurogenic cough has demonstrated benefit with reduction in the CSI [106, 107]

Further prospective studies are warranted to confirm the success of SLN block for the treatment of neurogenic cough, and the applicability to other causes of chronic cough would be of interest.

Deep Vocal Fold Injection Augmentation

The use of deep vocal fold injection augmentation to treat chronic cough was reported in 2015 by Crawley et al. [108]. This was a case series of six patients, among whom five reported improvement in CSI with this procedure. The selected patients had a diagnosis of vocal fold paresis as the suspected etiology of their chronic cough. Similarly, Litts et al. reported on their retrospective series of 23 patients with a diagnosis of glottic insufficiency, predominantly due to vocal fold atrophy (21/23 patients). A significant improvement in CSI was noted post-injection, but 11 patients reported recurrence of their symptom 4 months following injection (performed with carboxymethylcellulose or hyaluronic acid). Eight of these patients subsequently opted for permanent medialization procedures, and the results of this intervention remain to be reported [109].

Level of evidence	Conclusion
4	In patients with evidence of glottic insufficiency, deep vocal fold injection augmentation has resulted in temporary improvement in CSI [108]

Botulinum Toxin

Botulinum toxin type A (Botox-A) is a potent neurotoxin produced by the anaerobic bacterium *Clostridium botulinum*. This toxin results in chemodenervation at the presynaptic neuromuscular junction by inhibiting release of the neurotransmitter acetylcholine. The toxin can also work by inhibiting other neurologic signaling markers such as substance P and glutamate and by modulating sensory feedback loops.

The first report of using botulinum toxin for the treatment of chronic cough in adults was published in 2010 by Chu et al. This was a retrospective case series of four patients without any identifiable cause of cough on workup and with failed empiric treatments. These patients were treated with bilateral thyroarytenoid botulinum toxin injections, with a median of 7 injections (range 4–16) and mean dose of 4.0 units. All four patients reported significant relief of their cough [110].

Subsequently, Sasieta and colleagues retrospectively reported their results using botulinum toxin A at a tertiary care cough clinic for refractory chronic cough. Pre-injection workup and previously trialed medications and treatments were well outlined and documented. Their cohort consisted of 22 patients infected bilaterally into the thyroarytenoid muscles with Botox-A. Treatment success was defined as a 50% reduction or more of cough severity during a follow-up phone call 2 months post injection. Fifty percent

($n = 11/22$) of the patients met criteria for treatment success after one injection, with 73% ($n = 16/22$) reporting at least some improvement in their cough. Unfortunately, treatment effect was not sustained, and patients required additional treatment of Botox-A injection due to worsening cough. No patient reported complete and permanent resolution of cough at the last follow-up [111].

Level of evidence	Conclusion
4	EMG-guided bilateral thyroarytenoid muscle injection with botulinum toxin-A resulted in a temporary treatment response for approximately 50% of patients with refractory chronic cough [111]

Other Management Options

Cough Suppression Therapy

Cough suppression therapy can be used as a primary or an adjunctive treatment modality. After thorough review of the available RCTs for treatment of unexplained chronic cough, the American College of Chest Physicians Evidence-Based Clinical Practice Guidelines suggest behavioral therapy as a reliable treatment option after ruling out possible contributing factors of lung, sinus or GERD [57].

A single-blind RCT looked at symptom outcomes for 47 patients with chronic cough undergoing cough suppression therapy versus 50 patients with chronic cough who participated in healthy lifestyle education as a placebo treatment [112]. The cough suppression therapy consisted of four components including education about the nature of chronic cough, strategies to help reduce cough (e.g. cough avoidance behaviors, improving voicing efficiency, pursed lip breathing, and relaxed throat breathing), laryngeal hygiene, and psycho-education counselling to motivate patients to take control of their symptoms. Results indicated that the therapy group reported significantly improved symptom scores in all five areas of breathing, cough, voice, upper airway, and overall limitation, while the placebo group noted significant improvement in the areas of breathing, cough, and overall limitation. Symptom improvements were significantly higher for the treatment group compared to the placebo group, and 88% of the treatment group participants reported the therapy as successful compared to only 14% of the placebo group.

A second randomized controlled trial compared similar interventions with 34 participants in the cough suppression therapy group and 41 in the placebo group. Chamberlain Mitchel et al. found significantly increased improvement in primary outcome LCQ scores compared to the control group. Improvement in cough frequency measured by a 24-hour probe for the cough therapy group was also found [113]. The LCQ improvement was sustained for both groups at 3 months, but at that time there was no difference between groups.

Level of evidence	Conclusion
1	Cough suppression therapy significantly improved airway symptoms (including cough) when compared with placebo [112]
1	Patients completing cough suppression therapy seem to show more improvement in cough-related quality of life scores when compared to placebo groups [113]

Cough suppression therapy can also be used in conjunction with other medical management options. Vertigan et al. randomly assigned 40 patients to a combination of behavioral cough therapy in conjunction with the use of either pregabalin or placebo medication [64]. This study found significantly increased improvement in LCQ score with the combination of cough therapy and pregabalin. Improvement in cough was maintained after pregabalin was withdrawn. There was no difference between groups for improvement in cough frequency or cough sensitivity.

Level of evidence	Conclusion
1	Cough therapy in conjunction with medical management may enhance efficacy of behavioral treatment [64]

Interestingly, a Cochrane review of the available randomized controlled trials suggested that there is not enough evidence to draw any robust conclusions about the efficacy of behavioral therapy for unexplained chronic cough. Although a large number of studies were identified initially, they included only two RCTs for the final review. Endpoints varied between the studies, and there was a paucity of data, limiting their ability to draw definitive conclusions [114]. There are also no long-term outcomes for behavioral therapy reported in any studies.

Conclusion

Chronic cough remains a common and challenging problem, with vast overlap between many different systems and diseases. Evidence supports first identifying the most probable etiologies, and targeting their treatment specifically. When this is ineffective, a multitude of alternative options are available to trial, with varying levels of evidence supporting their utility and effectiveness. By following an algorithmic approach and employing treatments with the most robust evidence, improvement in chronic cough is achievable in the majority of patients. Higher quality studies should be designed to investigate therapeutic options with insufficient or low-quality evidence, and these management strategies should be reserved for when best-evidence treatment strategies fail.

References

1. Ford AC, Forman D, Moayyedi P, Morice AH. Cough in the community: a cross sectional survey and the relationship to gastrointestinal symptoms. Thorax. 2006;61(11):975–9.

2. Irwin RS, French CL, Chang AB, Altman KW, Panel* CEC. Classification of cough as a symptom in adults and management algorithms: CHEST guideline and expert panel report. Chest. 2018;153(1):196–209.
3. Canning BJ, Chang AB, Bolser DC, Smith JA, Mazzone SB, McGarvey L, et al. Anatomy and neurophysiology of cough: CHEST Guideline and Expert Panel report. Chest. 2014;146(6):1633–48.
4. Widdicombe J. Airway receptors. Respir Physiol. 2001;125(1–2):3–15.
5. Groneberg DA, Niimi A, Dinh QT, Cosio B, Hew M, Fischer A, et al. Increased expression of transient receptor potential vanilloid-1 in airway nerves of chronic cough. Am J Respir Crit Care Med. 2004;170(12):1276–80.
6. Coleridge JC, Coleridge HM. Afferent vagal C fibre innervation of the lungs and airways and its functional significance. Rev Physiol Biochem Pharmacol. 1984;99:1–110.
7. Lee LY, Pisarri TE. Afferent properties and reflex functions of bronchopulmonary C-fibers. Respir Physiol. 2001;125(1–2):47–65.
8. Undem BJ, Chuaychoo B, Lee MG, Weinreich D, Myers AC, Kollarik M. Subtypes of vagal afferent C-fibres in guinea-pig lungs. J Physiol. 2004;556(Pt 3):905–17.
9. Szallasi A, Blumberg PM. Vanilloid (Capsaicin) receptors and mechanisms. Pharmacol Rev. 1999;51(2):159–212.
10. Canning BJ, Mazzone SB, Meeker SN, Mori N, Reynolds SM, Undem BJ. Identification of the tracheal and laryngeal afferent neurones mediating cough in anaesthetized guinea-pigs. J Physiol. 2004;557(Pt 2):543–58.
11. Canning BJ, Chou YL. Cough sensors. I. Physiological and pharmacological properties of the afferent nerves regulating cough. Handb Exp Pharmacol. 2009;187:23–47.
12. Canning BJ. Afferent nerves regulating the cough reflex: mechanisms and mediators of cough in disease. Otolaryngol Clin N Am. 2010;43(1):15–25. vii
13. Canning BJ, Mazzone SB. Reflex mechanisms in gastroesophageal reflux disease and asthma. Am J Med. 2003;115 Suppl 3A:45S–8S.
14. Fox AJ, Lalloo UG, Belvisi MG, Bernareggi M, Chung KF, Barnes PJ. Bradykinin-evoked sensitization of airway sensory nerves: a mechanism for ACE-inhibitor cough. Nat Med. 1996;2(7):814–7.
15. Choudry NB, Fuller RW, Pride NB. Sensitivity of the human cough reflex: effect of inflammatory mediators prostaglandin E2, bradykinin, and histamine. Am Rev Respir Dis. 1989;140(1):137–41.
16. Nichol G, Nix A, Barnes PJ, Chung KF. Prostaglandin F2 alpha enhancement of capsaicin induced cough in man: modulation by beta 2 adrenergic and anticholinergic drugs. Thorax. 1990;45(9):694–8.
17. Israili ZH, Hall WD. Cough and angioneurotic edema associated with angiotensin-converting enzyme inhibitor therapy. A review of the literature and pathophysiology. Ann Intern Med. 1992;117(3):234–42.

18. Dicpinigaitis PV. Angiotensin-converting enzyme inhibitor-induced cough: ACCP evidence-based clinical practice guidelines. Chest. 2006;129(1 Suppl):169S–73S.

19. Irwin RS, Baumann MH, Bolser DC, Boulet LP, Braman SS, Brightling CE, et al. Diagnosis and management of cough executive summary: ACCP evidence-based clinical practice guidelines. Chest. 2006;129(1 Suppl):1S–23S.

20. Mello CJ, Irwin RS, Curley FJ. Predictive values of the character, timing, and complications of chronic cough in diagnosing its cause. Arch Intern Med. 1996;156(9):997–1003.

21. Irwin RS, Curley FJ, French CL. Chronic cough. The spectrum and frequency of causes, key components of the diagnostic evaluation, and outcome of specific therapy. Am Rev Respir Dis. 1990;141(3):640–7.

22. Pratter MR. Chronic upper airway cough syndrome secondary to rhinosinus diseases (previously referred to as postnasal drip syndrome): ACCP evidence-based clinical practice guidelines. Chest. 2006;129(1 Suppl):63S–71S.

23. Dworkin JP. Laryngitis: types, causes, and treatments. Otolaryngol Clin N Am. 2008;41(2):419–36. ix

24. Senior BA, Kennedy DW, Tanabodee J, Kroger H, Hassab M, Lanza DC. Long-term impact of functional endoscopic sinus surgery on asthma. Otolaryngol Head Neck Surg. 1999;121(1):66–8.

25. Morice AH, McGarvey L, Pavord I, British Thoracic Society Cough Guideline G. Recommendations for the management of cough in adults. Thorax. 2006;61 Suppl 1:i1–24.

26. Gawchik S, Goldstein S, Prenner B, John A. Relief of cough and nasal symptoms associated with allergic rhinitis by mometasone furoate nasal spray. Ann Allergy Asthma Immunol. 2003;90(4):416–21.

27. Pratter MR, Bartter T, Akers S, DuBois J. An algorithmic approach to chronic cough. Ann Intern Med. 1993;119(10):977–83.

28. Maxfield AZ, Bleier BS. Sinonasal disease and allergy as an etiology of chronic cough. In: Carroll CC, editor. Chronic cough. San Diego: Plural Publishing; 2019. p. 39–64.

29. Studham J, Fuller RW. The effect of oral terfenadine on the sensitivity of the cough reflex in normal volunteers. Pulm Pharmacol. 1992;5(1):51–2.

30. Dicpinigaitis PV, Spinner L, Santhyadka G, Negassa A. Effect of tiotropium on cough reflex sensitivity in acute viral cough. Lung. 2008;186(6):369–74.

31. McGarvey LP, Heaney L, Lawson JT, Johnston BT, Scally CM, Ennis M, Shepherd DR, MacMahon J. Evaluation and outcome of patients with chronic non-productive cough using a comprehensive diagnostic protocol. Thorax. 1998;53(9):738–43.

32. Macedo P, Saleh H, Torrego A, Arbery J, MacKay I, Durham SR, et al. Postnasal drip and chronic cough: an open interventional study. Respir Med. 2009;103(11):1700–5.

33. Holmes PW, Barter CE, Pierce RJ. Chronic persistent cough: use of ipratropium bromide in undiagnosed cases following upper respiratory tract infection. Respir Med. 1992;86(5):425–9.

34. Lowry R, Wood A, Higenbottam T. The effect of anticholinergic bronchodilator therapy on cough during upper respiratory tract infections. Br J Clin Pharmacol. 1994;37(2):187–91.

35. Harvey R, Hannan SA, Badia L, Scadding G. Nasal saline irrigations for the symptoms of chronic rhinosinusitis. Cochrane Database Syst Rev. 2007;(3):CD006394.

36. van den Berg JW, de Nier LM, Kaper NM, Schilder AG, Venekamp RP, Grolman W, et al. Limited evidence: higher efficacy of nasal saline irrigation over nasal saline spray in chronic rhinosinusitis – an update and reanalysis of the evidence base. Otolaryngol Head Neck Surg. 2014;150(1):16–21.

37. Pynnonen MA, Mukerji SS, Kim HM, Adams ME, Terrell JE. Nasal saline for chronic sinonasal symptoms: a randomized controlled trial. Arch Otolaryngol Head Neck Surg. 2007;133(11):1115–20.

38. Lin L, Chen Z, Cao Y, Sun G. Normal saline solution nasal-pharyngeal irrigation improves chronic cough associated with allergic rhinitis. Am J Rhinol Allergy. 2017;31(2):96–104.

39. Varshney R, Lee JT. Current trends in topical therapies for chronic rhinosinusitis: update and literature review. Expert Opin Drug Deliv. 2017;14(2):257–71.

40. Chiu AG, Palmer JN, Woodworth BA, Doghramji L, Cohen MB, Prince A, et al. Baby shampoo nasal irrigations for the symptomatic post-functional endoscopic sinus surgery patient. Am J Rhinol. 2008;22(1):34–7.

41. Scott JR, Krishnan R, Rotenberg BW, Sowerby LJ. The effectiveness of topical colloidal silver in recalcitrant chronic rhinosinusitis: a randomized crossover control trial. J Otolaryngol Head Neck Surg. 2017;46(1):64.

42. Neher A, Fischer H, Appenroth E, Lass-Florl C, Mayr A, Gschwendtner A, et al. Tolerability of N-chlorotaurine in chronic rhinosinusitis applied via yamik catheter. Auris Nasus Larynx. 2005;32(4):359–64.

43. Brigham EP, West NE. Diagnosis of asthma: diagnostic testing. Int Forum Allergy Rhinol. 2015;5 Suppl 1:S27–30.

44. Brightling CE, Pavord ID. Eosinophilic bronchitis: an important cause of prolonged cough. Ann Med. 2000;32(7):446–51.

45. Lai K, Chen R, Peng W, Zhan W. Non-asthmatic eosinophilic bronchitis and its relationship with asthma. Pulm Pharmacol Ther. 2017;47:66–71.

46. Irwin RS. Chronic cough due to gastroesophageal reflux disease: ACCP evidence-based clinical practice guidelines. Chest. 2006;129(1 Suppl):80S–94S.

47. Ours TM, Kavuru MS, Schilz RJ, Richter JE. A prospective evaluation of esophageal testing and a double-blind, randomized study of omeprazole in a diagnostic and therapeutic algorithm for chronic cough. Am J Gastroenterol. 1999;94(11):3131–8.

48. Kiljander TO, Salomaa ER, Hietanen EK, Terho EO. Chronic cough and gastro-oesophageal reflux: a double-blind placebo-controlled study with omeprazole. Eur Respir J. 2000;16(4):633–8.

49. Chang AB, Lasserson TJ, Gaffney J, Connor FL, Garske LA. Gastro-oesophageal reflux treatment for prolonged non-specific cough in children and adults. Cochrane Database Syst Rev. 2011;(1):CD004823.

50. Chang AB, Lasserson TJ, Gaffney J, Connor FL, Garske LA. Gastro-oesophageal reflux treatment for prolonged non-specific cough in children and adults. Cochrane Database Syst Rev. 2006;(4):CD004823.

51. Chang AB, Lasserson TJ, Kiljander TO, Connor FL, Gaffney JT, Garske LA. Systematic review and meta-analysis of randomised controlled trials of gastro-oesophageal reflux interventions for chronic cough associated with gastro-oesophageal reflux. BMJ. 2006;332(7532):11–7.

52. Kahrilas PJ, Altman KW, Chang AB, Field SK, Harding SM, Lane AP, et al. Chronic cough due to gastroesophageal reflux in adults: CHEST guideline and expert panel report. Chest. 2016;150(6):1341–60.

53. Kaufman JA, Houghland JE, Quiroga E, Cahill M, Pellegrini CA, Oelschlager BK. Long-term outcomes of laparoscopic antireflux surgery for gastroesophageal reflux disease (GERD)-related airway disorder. Surg Endosc. 2006;20(12):1824–30.

54. Drews G, Rudolph F, Martinenko O, Kuhne P, Schreiber J. [The influence of laparoscopic fundoplication on reflux-associated cough]. Zentralbl Chir. 2016;141(5):545–51.

55. Iqbal M, Batch AJ, Spychal RT, Cooper BT. Outcome of surgical fundoplication for extraesophageal (atypical) manifestations of gastroesophageal reflux disease in adults: a systematic review. J Laparoendosc Adv Surg Tech A. 2008;18(6):789–96.

56. Pavord ID, Chung KF. Management of chronic cough. Lancet. 2008;371(9621):1375–84.

57. Gibson P, Wang G, McGarvey L, Vertigan AE, Altman KW, Birring SS, et al. Treatment of unexplained chronic cough: CHEST guideline and expert panel report. Chest. 2016;149(1):27–44.

58. Altman KW, Noordzij JP, Rosen CA, Cohen S, Sulica L. Neurogenic cough. Laryngoscope. 2015;125(7):1675–81.

59. Chung KF, McGarvey L, Mazzone SB. Chronic cough as a neuropathic disorder. Lancet Respir Med. 2013;1(5):414–22.

60. Morrison M, Rammage L, Emami AJ. The irritable larynx syndrome. J Voice. 1999;13(3):447–55.

61. Amin MR, Koufman JA. Vagal neuropathy after upper respiratory infection: a viral etiology? Am J Otolaryngol. 2001;22(4):251–6.

62. Lee B, Woo P. Chronic cough as a sign of laryngeal sensory neuropathy: diagnosis and treatment. Ann Otol Rhinol Laryngol. 2005;114(4):253–7.

63. Jeyakumar A, Brickman TM, Haben M. Effectiveness of amitriptyline versus cough suppressants in the treatment of chronic cough resulting from postviral vagal neuropathy. Laryngoscope. 2006;116(12):2108–12.

64. Vertigan AE, Kapela SL, Ryan NM, Birring SS, McElduff P, Gibson PG. Pregabalin and speech pathology combination therapy for refractory chronic cough: a randomized controlled trial. Chest. 2016;149(3):639–48.

65. Ryan NM, Birring SS, Gibson PG. Gabapentin for refractory chronic cough: a randomised, double-blind, placebo-controlled trial. Lancet. 2012;380(9853):1583–9.

66. Bastian RW, Vaidya AM, Delsupehe KG. Sensory neuropathic cough: a common and treatable cause of chronic cough. Otolaryngol Head Neck Surg. 2006;135(1):17–21.

67. Norris BK, Schweinfurth JM. Management of recurrent laryngeal sensory neuropathic symptoms. Ann Otol Rhinol Laryngol. 2010;119(3):188–91.

68. Giliberto JP, Merati A. Neurogenic cough. In: Carroll CC, editor. Chronic cough. San Diego: Plural Publishing; 2019. p. 97–115.

69. Dion GR, Teng SE, Achlatis E, Fang Y, Amin MR. Treatment of neurogenic cough with tramadol: a pilot study. Otolaryngol Head Neck Surg. 2017;157(1):77–9.

70. Tjaderborn M, Jonsson AK, Ahlner J, Hagg S. Tramadol dependence: a survey of spontaneously reported cases in Sweden. Pharmacoepidemiol Drug Saf. 2009;18(12):1192–8.

71. Dicpinigaitis PV, Dobkin JB, Rauf K, Aldrich TK. Inhibition of capsaicin-induced cough by the gamma-aminobutyric acid agonist baclofen. J Clin Pharmacol. 1998;38(4):364–7.

72. Dicpinigaitis PV, Dobkin JB. Antitussive effect of the GABA-agonist baclofen. Chest. 1997;111(4):996–9.

73. Cohen SM, Misono S. Use of specific neuromodulators in the treatment of chronic, idiopathic cough: a systematic review. Otolaryngol Head Neck Surg. 2013;148(3):374–82.

74. Giliberto JP, Cohen SM, Misono S. Are neuromodulating medications effective for the treatment of chronic neurogenic cough? Laryngoscope. 2017;127(5):1007–8.

75. Pizzichini MM, Pizzichini E, Parameswaran K, Clelland L, Efthimiadis A, Dolovich J, et al. Nonasthmatic chronic cough: no effect of treatment with an inhaled corticosteroid in patients without sputum eosinophilia. Can Respir J. 1999;6(4):323–30.

76. Ribeiro M, Pereira CA, Nery LE, Beppu OS, Silva CO. High-dose inhaled beclomethasone treatment in patients with chronic cough: a randomized placebo-controlled study. Ann Allergy Asthma Immunol. 2007;99(1):61–8.

77. Chaudhuri R, McMahon AD, Thomson LJ, MacLeod KJ, McSharry CP, Livingston E, et al. Effect of inhaled corticosteroids on symptom severity and sputum mediator levels in chronic persistent cough. J Allergy Clin Immunol. 2004;113(6):1063–70.

78. Johnstone KJ, Chang AB, Fong KM, Bowman RV, Yang IA. Inhaled corticosteroids for subacute and chronic cough in adults. Cochrane Database Syst Rev. 2013;(3):CD009305.

79. Faruqi S, Molyneux ID, Fathi H, Wright C, Thompson R, Morice AH. Chronic cough and esomeprazole: a double-blind placebo-controlled parallel study. Respirology. 2011;16(7):1150–6.

80. Shaheen NJ, Crockett SD, Bright SD, Madanick RD, Buckmire R, Couch M, et al. Randomised clinical trial: high-dose acid suppression for chronic cough - a double-blind, placebo-controlled study. Aliment Pharmacol Ther. 2011;33(2):225–34.

81. Simpson JL, Powell H, Boyle MJ, Scott RJ, Gibson PG. Clarithromycin targets neutrophilic airway inflammation in refractory asthma. Am J Respir Crit Care Med. 2008;177(2):148–55.

82. Brusselle GG, Vanderstichele C, Jordens P, Deman R, Slabbynck H, Ringoet V, et al. Azithromycin for prevention of exacerbations in severe asthma (AZISAST): a multicentre randomised double-blind placebo-controlled trial. Thorax. 2013;68(4):322–9.

83. Seemungal TA, Wilkinson TM, Hurst JR, Perera WR, Sapsford RJ, Wedzicha JA. Long-term erythromycin therapy is associated with decreased chronic obstructive pulmonary disease exacerbations. Am J Respir Crit Care Med. 2008;178(11):1139–47.

84. Jatakanon A, Lalloo UG, Lim S, Chung KF, Barnes PJ. Increased neutrophils and cytokines, TNF-alpha and IL-8, in induced sputum of non-asthmatic patients with chronic dry cough. Thorax. 1999;54(3):234–7.

85. Yousaf N, Monteiro W, Parker D, Matos S, Birring S, Pavord ID. Long-term low-dose erythromycin in patients with unexplained chronic cough: a double-blind placebo controlled trial. Thorax. 2010;65(12):1107–10.

86. Hodgson D, Anderson J, Reynolds C, Oborne J, Meakin G, Bailey H, et al. The effects of azithromycin in treatment-resistant cough: a randomized, double-blind, placebo-controlled trial. Chest. 2016;149(4):1052–60.

87. Hay AD, Little P, Harnden A, Thompson M, Wang K, Kendrick D, et al. Effect of oral prednisolone on symptom duration and severity in non-asthmatic adults with acute lower respiratory tract infection: a randomized clinical trial. JAMA. 2017;318(8):721–30.

88. Raeessi MA, Aslani J, Raeessi N, Gharaie H, Karimi Zarchi AA, Raeessi F. Honey plus coffee versus systemic steroid in the treatment of persistent post-infectious cough: a randomised controlled trial. Prim Care Respir J. 2013;22(3):325–30.

89. Yancy WS Jr, McCrory DC, Coeytaux RR, Schmit KM, Kemper AR, Goode A, et al. Efficacy and tolerability of treatments for chronic cough: a systematic review and meta-analysis. Chest. 2013;144(6):1827–38.

90. Woodcock A, McLeod RL, Sadeh J, Smith JA. The efficacy of a NOP1 agonist (SCH486757) in subacute cough. Lung. 2010;188(Suppl 1):S47–52.

91. Morice AH, Menon MS, Mulrennan SA, Everett CF, Wright C, Jackson J, et al. Opiate therapy in chronic cough. Am J Respir Crit Care Med. 2007;175(4):312–5.

92. Matthys H, Bleicher B, Bleicher U. Dextromethorphan and codeine: objective assessment of antitussive activity in patients with chronic cough. J Int Med Res. 1983;11(2):92–100.

93. Fuller RW, Dixon CM, Barnes PJ. Bronchoconstrictor response to inhaled capsaicin in humans. J Appl Physiol (1985). 1985;58(4):1080–4.

94. Chung KF. Chronic 'cough hypersensitivity syndrome': a more precise label for chronic cough. Pulm Pharmacol Ther. 2011;24(3):267–71.

95. Vertigan AE, Gibson PG. Chronic refractory cough as a sensory neuropathy: evidence from a reinterpretation of cough triggers. J Voice. 2011;25(5):596–601.

96. Morice AH, Millqvist E, Belvisi MG, Bieksiene K, Birring SS, Chung KF, et al. Expert opinion on the cough hypersensitivity syndrome in respiratory medicine. Eur Respir J. 2014;44(5):1132–48.

97. Ternesten-Hasseus E, Johansson EL, Millqvist E. Cough reduction using capsaicin. Respir Med. 2015;109(1):27–37.

98. Fukumitsu K, Kanemitsu Y, Asano T, Takeda N, Ichikawa H, Yap JMG, et al. Tiotropium attenuates refractory cough and capsaicin cough reflex sensitivity in patients with asthma. J Allergy Clin Immunol Pract. 2018;6(5):1613–20. e2

99. Birrell MA, Bonvini SJ, Dubuis E, Maher SA, Wortley MA, Grace MS, et al. Tiotropium modulates transient receptor potential V1 (TRPV1) in airway sensory nerves: a beneficial off-target effect? J Allergy Clin Immunol. 2014;133(3):679–87. e9

100. Zanasi A, Lecchi M, Del Forno M, Fabbri E, Mastroroberto M, Mazzolini M, et al. A randomized, placebo-controlled, double-blind trial on the management of post-infective cough by inhaled ipratropium and salbutamol administered in combination. Pulm Pharmacol Ther. 2014;29(2):224–32.

101. Kwong K, Kollarik M, Nassenstein C, Ru F, Undem BJ. P2X2 receptors differentiate placodal vs. neural crest C-fiber phenotypes innervating guinea pig lungs and esophagus. Am J Physiol Lung Cell Mol Physiol. 2008;295(5):L858–65.

102. Weigand LA, Ford AP, Undem BJ. A role for ATP in bronchoconstriction-induced activation of guinea pig vagal intrapulmonary C-fibres. J Physiol. 2012;590(16):4109–20.

103. Abdulqawi R, Dockry R, Holt K, Layton G, McCarthy BG, Ford AP, et al. P2X3 receptor antagonist (AF-219) in refractory chronic cough: a randomised, double-blind, placebo-controlled phase 2 study. Lancet. 2015;385(9974):1198–205.

104. Khalid S, Murdoch R, Newlands A, Smart K, Kelsall A, Holt K, et al. Transient receptor potential vanilloid 1 (TRPV1) antagonism in patients with refractory chronic cough: a double-blind randomized controlled trial. J Allergy Clin Immunol. 2014;134(1):56–62.

105. Belvisi MG, Birrell MA, Wortley MA, Maher SA, Satia I, Badri H, et al. XEN-D0501, a novel transient receptor potential Vanilloid 1 antagonist, does not reduce cough in patients with refractory cough. Am J Respir Crit Care Med. 2017;196(10):1255–63.

106. Simpson CB, Tibbetts KM, Loochtan MJ, Dominguez LM. Treatment of chronic neurogenic cough with in-office superior laryngeal nerve block. Laryngoscope. 2018;128(8):1898–903.

107. Dhillon VK. Superior laryngeal nerve block for neurogenic cough: a case series. Laryngoscope Investig Otolaryngol. 2019;4(4):410–3.

108. Crawley BK, Murry T, Sulica L. Injection augmentation for chronic cough. J Voice. 2015;29(6):763–7.

109. Litts JK, Fink DS, Clary MS. The effect of vocal fold augmentation on cough symptoms in the presence of glottic insufficiency. Laryngoscope. 2018;128(6):1316–9.

110. Chu MW, Lieser JD, Sinacori JT. Use of botulinum toxin type A for chronic cough: a neuropathic model. Arch Otolaryngol Head Neck Surg. 2010;136(5):447–52.

111. Sasieta HC, Iyer VN, Orbelo DM, Patton C, Pittelko R, Keogh K, et al. Bilateral thyroarytenoid botulinum toxin type A injection for the treatment of refractory chronic cough. JAMA Otolaryngol Head Neck Surg. 2016;142(9):881–8.

112. Vertigan AE, Theodoros DG, Gibson PG, Winkworth AL. Efficacy of speech pathology management for chronic cough: a randomised placebo controlled trial of treatment efficacy. Thorax. 2006;61(12):1065–9.

113. Chamberlain Mitchell SA, Garrod R, Clark L, Douiri A, Parker SM, Ellis J, et al. Physiotherapy, and speech and language therapy intervention for patients with refractory chronic cough: a multicentre randomised control trial. Thorax. 2017;72(2):129–36.

114. Slinger C, Mehdi SB, Milan SJ, Dodd S, Matthews J, Vyas A, et al. Speech and language therapy for management of chronic cough. Cochrane Database Syst Rev. 2019;7:CD013067.

Laryngotracheal Stenosis

8

David E. Rosow, Debbie R. Pan,
and James W. Bao

Introduction

Laryngotracheal stenosis (LTS) refers to a heterogeneous set of conditions in which the airway is narrowed at the level of the supraglottis, glottis, subglottis, or trachea, resulting in potentially life-threatening restriction in ventilation. Due to its relative rarity but commonplace symptoms, LTS can be a difficult disease to diagnose and treat. Patients may present with a range of respiratory symptoms, including wheezing, shortness of breath, hoarseness, stridor, exertional dyspnea, and asphyxiation [1]. While surgical and nonsurgical management have been beneficial for many cases, clinical outcomes vary in success and need for long-term management. A major factor in management is the recurrent nature of the disease, which may result in repeated surgeries and

D. E. Rosow (✉) · J. W. Bao
Department of Otolaryngology, University of Miami Miller School of Medicine, Miami, FL, USA
e-mail: DRosow@med.miami.edu

D. R. Pan
Department of Head and Neck Surgery & Communication Sciences, Duke University, Durham, NC, USA

© Springer Nature Switzerland AG 2021
D. E. Rosow, C. M. Ivey (eds.), *Evidence-Based Laryngology*,
https://doi.org/10.1007/978-3-030-58494-8_8

hospital stays. As research continues to elucidate the specific pathogenesis, risk factors, and proper therapies for different cases of LTS, there is promising potential for more strategic, preventative, and personalized treatment strategies for patients.

The majority of cases of LTS result from intubation and tracheostomy (iatrogenic), but the condition has also been shown to arise from trauma, infection, neoplasm, autoimmune disorders, and idiopathic causes [2]. Incidence of post-intubation adult LTS is about 1 in 200,000 patients per year, with the subglottic region being the most commonly affected area [3]. There can be misdiagnosis rates in as high as 80% of patients, with LTS frequently classified as asthma and other pulmonary disorders [4, 5]. Also, delays in diagnosis can take up to 18 months, which increases risk of treatment failure, respiratory complications, and morbidity [6]. Treatment of LTS mostly includes surgical intervention to reopen and maintain the airway, with approaches that include arytenoidectomy, posterior cordectomy, endoscopic dilation, open tracheal resection, and tracheostomy. Some nonsurgical adjuvant therapies such as mitomycin C, methotrexate, and corticosteroids have also shown efficacy. In this chapter, we will provide a discussion of the most current research with evidence of successful outcomes demonstrating improvements in symptoms, disease burden, and quality of life.

Etiology and Pathophysiology

In a retrospective cohort study of 150 adult LTS patients by Gelbard et al., 54.7% had an iatrogenic etiology and the remaining 45.3% were either traumatic, autoimmune, or idiopathic [2]. According to Stauffer et al., approximately 10% of prospectively studied intubated patients developed LTS [7]. Regardless of the specific etiology, the defining factors in the pathogenesis of LTS are inflammation, necrosis, and fibrosis of the airway.

For iatrogenic cases, it has been suggested that prolonged intubation causes the initial tissue injury and blood vessel compromise that leads to local ischemia and scar formation [8]. Increased cases of LTS have been linked to an improper endotracheal tube size. Airway size differs depending on factors such as gender and obesity, and a reduced airway diameter has been shown to increase risk of LTS. In the study by Gelbard et al., 83% of healthy iatrogenic LTS patients without other comorbidities such as obesity, type 2 diabetes mellitus (DMII), and cardiovascular disease were women. The authors suggest this may be due to the smaller airway size of women compared to men [2].

Level of evidence	Conclusion
4	83% of healthy iatrogenic LTS patients are women, suggesting the contributory role of reduced airway diameter to increased risk [2]

In a multicenter retrospective study of airway complications in tracheostomy patients by Halum et al., the use of large endotracheal tubes (>7.5 mm in diameter) was correlated with an increased rate of LTS, particularly in obese patients [9]. 9.9% of obese patients developed stenosis post-intubation with a tube size >7.5 mm. In contrast, only 0.4% of non-obese patients developed stenosis under the same intubation conditions. Furthermore, in obese patients who were intubated with tubes <7.5 mm, the rate of stenosis dropped to 1.9%. As for total cases of stenosis, significantly more obese individuals developed LTS than non-obese individuals because obese individuals were more often intubated with larger tubes. Over 45% of obese patients were intubated with 8.0 mm tubes, whereas a little over 30% of non-obese patients were intubated with these sizes. Therefore, both obesity and endotracheal tube size appear to increase risk of developing LTS [9].

Level of evidence	Conclusion
4	Obesity and large endotracheal tube size increase the risk of developing LTS after endotracheal intubation [9]

Stenosis can also occur from external trauma, such as from motor vehicle accidents, with resulting cartilaginous fractures and mucosal tears. Internal trauma, in addition to trauma from intubation, can arise from chemical or thermal burns. Other iatrogenic causes include laryngotracheal surgery or irradiation, which can cause edema and necrosis of tissue. Infections such as syphilis, diphtheria, tuberculosis, aspergillus, and others can cause granuloma formation and scarring [10]. In addition, multiple series have also shown that DMII makes patients particularly vulnerable to tracheal injury and LTS development [2, 11]. Gadkaree et al. suggests this is due to impaired mucosal wound healing in DMII patients, exacerbated by intubation-associated injury. This same series concluded that other comorbidities promoting microvascular injury, such as chronic smoking and chronic obstructive pulmonary disease (COPD), led to increased prevalence of iatrogenic LTS [11].

Level of evidence	Conclusion
4	There is an increased prevalence of iatrogenic LTS in patients with DMII, smoking, and COPD due to increased risk of microvascular injury [11]

LTS of autoimmune origin is an interesting subtype linked most commonly to Wegener's granulomatosis, now more commonly called granulomatosis with polyangiitis (GPA). GPA is a rare systemic inflammatory disease presenting with necrotizing granulomatous inflammation and small or medium vessel vasculitis in the respiratory tract and kidneys [12]. Only a small percentage of patients with GPA have associated LTS (8–23% according to Dablanca et al.), but other autoimmune disorders are also associated with LTS, making LTS of autoimmune etiology the fifth most common subtype. In a retrospective study by Dablanca et al., four out of nine patients with autoimmune LTS had GPA; the remaining cases were diagnosed with unspecified vasculitis and elevated antinuclear antibodies [13]. The etiology of GPA is unknown, but it is hypothesized that anti-neutrophil cytoplasmic antibodies (ANCA) activate neutrophils and induce inflammation, which degrades cartilage and exposes type II collagen to the immune system, leading to further inflammation and eventual stenosis [13].

In cases where there is no clear source of trauma or inflammation, patients are diagnosed with idiopathic LTS, most commonly arising in the subglottis. Idiopathic subglottic stenosis (iSGS) is rare, but recent studies have elucidated several pathways that could promote the disease. Idiopathic SGS is associated with extensive fibrotic remodeling, especially at the laryngotracheal transition [14]. One possible cause is gastroesophageal reflux (GER), specifically laryngopharyngeal reflux (LPR), as an instigator in the abnormal response to injury of the laryngotracheal epithelium and the chronic inflammation needed for LTS. In a prospective cohort study by Koufman et al., 78% of LTS patients had abnormal pH findings indicative of GER (pH < 4), and 56% had abnormal pharyngeal reflux [15]. In a similar study by Maronian et al., 12 out of 14 patients with subglottic stenosis had pH <4 at the laryngeal level, demonstrating an association between LPR and subglottic stenosis [16].

Level of evidence	Conclusion
3	Signs of LPR are often found in patients with LTS, indicating a possible association between reflux and stenosis [15, 16]

The proposed mechanism for the scarring that occurs in LTS occurs in the epithelial to mesenchymal transition (EMT) of the airway. In a translational research study by Aldhahrani et al., cultured human primary tracheal epithelial cells incubated with bile acids showed decreased epithelial markers (E-cadherin) and increased mesenchymal markers (fibronectin, matrix metalloproteinase-9, procollagen), supporting the theory that bile acids induce EMT in airway epithelium [17]. In contrast, pepsin, another component of reflux, was shown to not have any effect on the EMT markers. Though pepsin is found at significant levels in the airway of patients with subglottic stenosis, it does not seem to have a direct role in EMT and fibrosis [18].

Pro-inflammatory interleukin pathways have also been studied to uncover the underlying inflammatory causes of LTS and iSGS. In histological samples from iSGS patients, Gelbard et al. found upregulated IL-17A, its upstream driver IL-23, and IL-1ß [14]. The IL-17A/IL-23 pathway is thought to have a role in the chronic inflammation in iSGS when dysregulated. IL-17A has also been linked to other fibrotic lung diseases such as obliterative bronchiolitis [19]. When fibroblasts derived from iSGS patients were cultured in the presence of IL-17A, they proliferated at a dose-dependent rate while control fibroblasts did not. Also, when scar fibroblasts were cultured with IL-17A, they produced pro-inflammatory chemokines and cytokines [20]. Interestingly, this study also found that there was no evidence of EMT or its markers, which contradicts the idea proposed in other recent research, so perhaps fibroblasts have a dominant role in inflammation and fibrosis in LTS [20]. Antagonists to the IL-1 receptor have been shown to inhibit early granulation formation in mouse laryngotracheal complexes [21]. In addition, most of the cells expressing IL-17A in the iSGS samples were γ/δ TCR+ cells, which could indicate that iSGS has an infectious origin. In a study by Hillel et al., researchers showed differences between the microbiota in scar tissue and surrounding tissue, as well as between different etiologies of LTS. Idiopathic LTS demonstrated increased *Mycobacterium, Moraxella,* and *Acinetobacter* [22]. *Moraxella* and *Acinetobacter* are known inflammatory pathogens in the respiratory system and can add to the association between pathogens and inflammation in idiopathic LTS.

Diagnosis

Diagnosis of LTS involves thorough history, physical, endoscopic and radiographic assessments of the laryngotracheal region. Careful attention should be given to history of recent intubation, laryngotracheal surgeries, internal and external trauma to the airway, autoimmune diseases, neoplasms, radiation, and other inflammatory diseases. Endoscopic evaluation is the primary preoperative step in LTS workup and its aims include determining the proximal and distal borders of the stenosis, narrowest airway lumen diameter, vocal fold involvement, presence of active inflammation, and stenosis characteristics (fresh/incipient vs. mature/cicatricial) [1, 10, 23]. Endoscopy can be done with several different techniques. Transnasal fiberoptic laryngoscopy (TNFL) can be done either awake or under anesthesia depending on the circumstances for the patient. Direct transoral laryngoscopy with rigid telescope or suspension microlaryngoscopy can be used to assess the exact location, length and degree of the stenosis, with the capability of recording real-time videos. Suspension microlaryngoscopy is especially useful for vocal fold assessment because it allows the physician to use retractors and probes to move the vocal folds and the cricoarytenoid joints. This helps to differentiate between posterior glottic stenosis and bilateral vocal fold paralysis, which is more easily spread apart by a retractor. Finally, bronchoesophagoscopy can be used to assess the lower airways and esophagus for further stenosis and inflammation [24]. Using this information, the stenosis can be classified using the following systems.

Firstly, stenosis is classified by which regions of the airway it encompasses. The airway in LTS is usually separated into supraglottic, glottic, subglottic, and tracheal regions. Classification is further categorized by stenosis severity. The most common classification system is the Myer-Cotton system devised in 1994. It organizes the severity of the stenotic region(s) into four grades, as shown below [25].

Myer-Cotton grade	% Obstruction of lumen
Grade I	≤50%
Grade II	51–70%
Grade III	71–99%
Grade IV	No detectable lumen

This system was originally devised for pediatric patients by determining the largest endotracheal tube that could be passed safely through the stenosis to the subglottis while comparing to the expected normal airway size. It has since been applied to adult LTS patients as well, with increases in grade corresponding to increases in disease severity and poorer outcomes. While most classification is done using the Myer-Cotton system, these grades may be too simplistic for adult LTS. Monnier et al. proposes that a letter (a, b, c, or d) be added to the Myer-Cotton classification to indicate how many regions are stenotic; "a" indicating one region and "d" indicating four regions [24]. Other classification systems such as McCaffrey and Lano are used less frequently but are described below as they are sometimes encountered in research [2].

	McCaffrey stages	Lano stages
Stage I	Subglottis or trachea, <1 cm	One subsite involvement
Stage II	Subglottis, >1 cm	Two subsite involvement
Stage III	Subglottis and trachea, >1 cm	Three subsite involvement
Stage IV	Any lesion involving glottis	

Additional assessments such as lung function tests, EKGs, neurological exam, 24-hour impedance pH test, and serologic exams can help uncover etiology of the stenosis, rule out other diagnoses, and determine severity of the condition. Spirometry assesses dyspnea severity and monitors respiratory function throughout treatment. Nouraei et al. studied the utility of expiratory disproportion index (EDI) calculated from spirometry data and determined that EDI can reliably diagnose LTS over other nonstenotic causes of respiratory distress such as asthma [4].

Level of evidence	Conclusion
3	Expiratory disproportion index (EDI) can reliably diagnose LTS as the source of respiratory symptoms [4]

24-hour pH testing is diagnostic for GER and LPR, depending on the location of the probe. Serological testing can help diagnose autoimmune LTS, but according to Hall et al., such testing only proved to be significant for positive ANCA in patients with GPA causing LTS [26].

Surgical Management

Arytenoidectomy/Posterior Cordotomy

Treatment of posterior glottic stenosis involves resection and reconstruction of the glottis. Two main procedures currently utilized are arytenoidectomy and posterior cordotomy, both of which can be done endoscopically. Posterior cordotomy involves unilateral or bilateral incision or resection of a wedge from the stenotic vocal fold near the posterior commissure. Arytenoidectomy involves ablation of the anteromedial part of the arytenoid cartilage and lateralization of the vocal fold [27, 28]. Both procedures effectively widen the posterior glottis to improve the patient's ability to breathe. The current surgical procedures utilize endoscopic lasers to vaporize tissue and cartilage. The CO_2 laser was first used as an alternative to endoscopic dilation and open tracheal resection. According to Dedo et al., endoscopic dilation was only effective for less severe cases of LTS, and open resection was too dramatic an intervention for a patient with only moderately severe LTS [29]. Endoscopic laser surgery provided a middle ground between the two procedures and proved to be reasonably effective. Eight out of 9 patients with glottic stenosis were successfully relieved of dyspnea and decannulated (if tracheotomy was present), while 2 patients needed revision; 9 out of 10 patients with subglottic or tracheal stenosis were also treated successfully [29].

Level of evidence	Conclusion
4	8/9 patients with posterior glottic stenosis and 9/10 patients with subglottic or tracheal stenosis were relieved of dyspnea and decannulated using CO_2 laser [29]

Dennis et al. introduced the use of CO_2 lasers to posterior cordotomy. In the six patients treated, all experienced relief of dyspnea, increased exercise tolerance, and subjectively "good" to "excellent" voice quality [30]. In a retrospective analysis, Riffat et al. showed that, out of 34 patients receiving CO_2 laser arytenoidectomy, posterior cordotomy or both, all ended treatment with adequate airway caliber, a 100% decannulation rate, and no complications besides two lip injuries and one dental injury. Four patients needed a second revision, but each resulted in successful outcomes [31].

Level of evidence	Conclusion
4	Arytenoidectomy and posterior cordotomy can be conducted with a CO_2 laser. Results from one series showed 100% success with 4 revisions needed [31]

Endoscopic Nd:YAG lasers can also be used for treatment of LTS. It can be applied to both rigid and flexible bronchoscopes. Leventhal et al. utilized a Nd:YAG laser on a flexible bronchoscope to treat patients with subglottic stenosis and produced 81% success [32]. Earlier studies by Ciccone et al. and Mehta et al. used rigid bronchoscopes to obtain a 100% success rate and a 71% success rate, respectively, though sample sizes were small [33, 34].

Level of evidence	Conclusion
4	Success in treatment of subglottic stenosis has ranged from 71% to 100% using Nd:YAG laser [32–34]

Nd:YAG laser used specifically for arytenoidectomy and posterior cordotomy has also shown success. Anand et al. utilized a Nd:YAG laser on seven patients with bilateral vocal fold abductor paralysis by performing arytenoidectomies and posterior cordotomies. All patients were decannulated and had subjectively adequate voice quality with no complications [35]. Nd:YAG lasers may have some advantages over CO_2 lasers, including better hemostatic ability, better precision, and shorter operative time [35]. However, the predominant modality of choice would still appear to be CO_2 based on the numerous publications describing this procedure.

New studies have used plasma field coblation as an alternative to laser ablation. Hu et al. demonstrated successful arytenoidectomies using coblation on 14 patients with glottic stenosis, with only one patient needing a revision [36]. Laser surgery is mostly safe and effective, but careful attention must be given as it can also cause burns to the upper airway and lungs. Coblation lowers the risk of complications because it works at a much lower temperature than lasers, damages less surrounding tissue, induces less intraoperative bleeding and postoperative pain, and provides a shorter recovery time; however, it is also less precise, more expensive, and more difficult to use in the trachea [36]. Although there is a lack of direct comparison between the two modalities, coblation has been gaining momentum in current otolaryngologic practice.

Level of evidence	Conclusion
4	Laryngoscopic coblation arytenoidectomy was successful in treating 14 glottic stenosis patients and may produce less complications than laser arytenoidectomy [36]

It is important to note that endoscopic surgery may not be the best procedure for every patient. Monnier et al. reviewed 100 cases where LTS patients were treated only endoscopically with a CO_2 or Nd:YAG laser. Results showed that endoscopic surgery was very effective for stenosis of Myer-Cotton grade I (92% return to near-normal airway luminal size). Success subsequently decreased significantly between grades, with 46% for grade II and 13% for grade III [37]. Compared to open surgery results for more severe cases, relief of dyspnea and decannulation was much greater in open surgeries than in endoscopic surgeries. While less severe cases of LTS can be treated conservatively with endoscopic procedures and the most severe cases with open surgery, there is greater ambiguity concerning which procedure to perform for LTS grades II and III. Monnier et al. provides the following criteria for endoscopic and open surgery [37].

Endoscopic surgery	Open surgery
Grade I subglottic stenosis	Grade II, III, and IV subglottic
Some grade II and mild grade III	stenosis
subglottic stenosis	Cartilaginous stenosis
Length of stenosis <1.5 cm	Loss of cartilage support
Membranous glottic web	Length of stenosis >1.5 cm
Interarytenoid adhesion	Posterior glottic stenosis with
Posterior glottic stenosis without	cricoarytenoid joint fixation[a]
cricoarytenoid joint fixation[a]	

[a]If there is cricoarytenoid fixation, endoscopic arytenoidectomy and posterior cordotomy can be fairly effective [37]

In fact, endoscopic surgery may need to be done more than once to optimize treatment. Failure of endoscopic surgery to alleviate stenosis or recurrence of stenosis to preoperative conditions (or worse) indicates the usage of open surgery instead [37].

Endoscopic Dilation

Endoscopic dilation is a procedure used frequently for the initial management of LTS and the maintenance of airway patency. It involves physical dilation of the airway, generally using either rigid dilators such as bronchoscopes and metal laryngeal dilators, or a radial expansion balloon catheter, which has become increasingly popular [1, 38, 39]. This usually includes making radial incisions using laser or coblation in the areas of stenosis to assist in the dilation [39]. In a retrospective review by Herrington et al. of 99 patients who underwent primary endoscopic dilation, 12 were cured and stenosis did not recur, but 37 went on to require open surgery [38]. Severity grades were not given for these patients, so while dilation is commonly effective, these cases may be representative of more severe stenosis. In a retrospective study of pediatric patients by Maresh et al., 14 out of 27 children were successfully treated for subglottic stenosis with only balloon dilation. Ten of these patients were grade II and four were grade III. All 13 that failed initial balloon dilation and needed subsequent laryngotracheoplasty were grade III [40].

Level of evidence	Conclusion
4	Successful endoscopic balloon dilation was observed in mostly grade II LTS patients, while grade III patients tended to need open surgery [40]

Number of dilations needed and time between dilations tend to vary from patient to patient. In a retrospective review of adult patients by Hseu et al., 45% needed only one dilation while 55% needed multiple dilations [39]. Meta-analysis of pediatric subglottic stenosis cases by Lange and Brietzke showed that mean number of dilations for each study was between 1 and 4.27 with a mean of 1.9, and success of primary balloon dilation ranged between 54% and 100% [41]. The average time between dilations, or time between disease recurrence, was reported to be 13.7 months by Hseu et al. and 10.5 months by Sinacori et al. [39, 42]. Interestingly, Sinacori et al. noted that the recurrence rate for patients with DMII was only 3.9 months.

Level of evidence	Conclusion
4	Average time between dilations ranges between 10.5 to 13.7 months [39, 42]

Additionally, voice outcomes for successful endoscopic dilations are generally favorable. Dilation improves subjective voice measures such as voice-related quality of life (V-RQOL) and grade, roughness, breathiness, asthenia, strain (GRBAS) and decreases total voice handicap index [43, 44]. Outcomes were worse in patients with multilevel stenosis than patients with single-level stenosis [1].

Level of evidence	Conclusion
4	Endoscopic dilation has been shown to improve voice outcomes, especially in single-level stenosis [43, 44]

There is currently a dichotomy between endoscopic dilation and open procedures, particularly in which situations each should be used and how successful post-treatment outcomes will be. In a systematic review of research by Lewis et al., 466 patients received initial open laryngotracheal resection and anastomosis and 101 patients received endoscopic procedures (dilation or resection) [45]. Patients who received open surgery presented with less need for additional surgery than those who received endoscopic procedures (32% vs. 44%) and presented with higher decannulation rates (89% vs. 63%) [45]. Yamamoto et al. report a success rate for adult endoscopic procedures across six studies between 40% and 82% [46]. However, endoscopic treatment is less morbid, has shorter operative times, and presents with less complications. Many studies report no major complications in endoscopic dilation [39–41] while one pediatric study reported 2 tracheal lacerations and 1 death [41]. Endoscopic dilation can even be done in an outpatient setting with minimally increased risk of complications compared to an inpatient setting. A case review by Hsu et al. determined that only 2.6% of LTS patients treated with endoscopic dilation over 10 years presented with postoperative complications and needed to be readmitted. There were no deaths associated with the procedure [47].

Level of evidence	Conclusion
4	Endoscopic dilation is low risk for complications in children and adults, even in the outpatient setting [39–41, 47].

Furthermore, the timing of when to best initiate endoscopic dilations is also debated among otolaryngologists. Initial treatment with dilation appears to work well in patients with grade I or II stenosis. Yamamoto et al. concluded that endoscopic treatment can be useful as a first attempt for stenosis with length <1 cm without framework destruction and Sinacori et al. concluded that it was most effective for stenosis limited to one region [42, 46]. However, if endoscopic treatment fails after the first or second attempt, it is often contraindicated to continue attempting endoscopic intervention in the same patient as it might worsen the existing stenosis [46].

Open Tracheal Resections

In patients with severe stenosis who do not experience relief with less invasive treatment options, open tracheal surgery may be explored. There are two main approaches: complete resection with end-to-end re-anastomosis or laryngotracheoplasty, which often involves the widening of the airway with cartilage grafting and placement of a temporary stent [1]. Certain factors suggest earlier consideration for open surgical intervention. These include multiple prior endoscopic dilations with recurrent stenosis, grade III or IV stenosis, disorganized scar formation, long segments of stenosis (>1 cm vertical length), or patient preference [48, 49]. While potential risks exist to injuring nearby structures including the vocal folds, recurrent laryngeal nerves, esophagus, and/or mediastinal vessels, tracheal resection and laryngotracheoplasty have shown to offer positive overall results as long-term management options.

In a meta-analysis by Yamamoto et al., the pooled success rate (defined as no further treatments required for laryngotracheal stenosis) for laryngotracheal resection and anastomosis from 12 retrospective studies was 95%, compared to laryngotracheoplasty from seven studies with 76% and endoscopic dilation with laser resection from six studies with success rates varying between 40% and 82% [46]. Each study examined a minimum of ten cases of laryngotracheal stenosis and composite meta-regression showed a significant difference in success rates between laryngotracheal resection and laryngotracheoplasty or endoscopic dilations. Furthermore, Wang et al. retrospectively examined 263 patients with idiopathic subglottic stenosis, of which 70% had undergone prior endoscopic intervention, who were treated with resection and reconstruction over a 42-year span and reported that 96% of patients did not require reoperation or tracheostomy placement post-surgery [50].

Level of evidence	Conclusion
4	Multiple case series report a success rate of 95–96% for definitive treatment of laryngotracheal stenosis by surgical resection and re-anastomosis [46, 50]

Several complications should be considered during preoperative counseling of patients electing to undergo open surgical intervention. Although reported rates are as low as 2.4% in one study, signs of anastomotic complications after tracheal resection should be carefully monitored. Findings as subtle as wound infection or mild tachycardia could be benign or could portend a complication as severe as anastomotic separation [51]. According to a multivariable analysis performed by Wright et al., several statistically significant risk factors, listed below, were identified to increase the odds of anastomotic complications such as granulation, stenosis, or separation, for patients undergoing tracheal resection [52]. These patients with complications were treated with either multiple endoscopic dilations (3%), temporary (21%) or permanent (27%) T-tube stents, temporary (9%) or permanent (19%) tracheostomies, or reoperation (21%) [52].

Level of evidence	Conclusion
3	Risk factors for anastomotic complications following tracheal resection include: reoperation, diabetes, lengthy resections (≥4 cm), laryngotracheal resection, age ≤17 years, preoperative tracheostomy [52]

Voice and swallowing changes may also be post-surgical manifestations as laryngotracheal resection technique can often depend on the site and extent of stenosis and baseline function of the vocal folds. For example, in subglottic stenosis, a cricotracheal approach is commonly undertaken in which partial resection of the cricoid can cause disruption of cricothyroid muscle attachment and result in lowering of pitch and difficulty with voice projection [53]. According to one study, normal voice was preserved in 45% of patients with subglottic stenosis after laryngotracheal resection and the remaining patients self-reported voice changes, of which failure to project their voice was the most common complaint [50]. However, despite these drawbacks, patients have demonstrated significant satisfaction with surgical treatment. In a study with 160 survey participants, patients reported being significantly more satisfied with outcomes after tracheal resection (76%) compared to other treatment options without resection (39%) [6]. Likewise, another survey with 180 participants who underwent laryngotracheal resection and reconstruction reported satisfaction, effectiveness, and symptom improvement as 9.4/10 on average for each [50]. In Lennon et al., all patients who underwent open airway reconstruction were able to return to their preoperative diet, but patients with temporary airway stents placed had longer dysphagia symptoms than those without stents [54].

Level of evidence	Conclusion
4	Patients with laryngotracheal stenosis self-report high levels of satisfaction with surgical resections [6, 50]

In addition to patient satisfaction, the burden of cost should also be discussed as this is another great consideration in quality of life. Recently published, Yin et al. described the first study to examine health care costs of adult laryngotracheal stenosis comparing open reconstruction (cricotracheal/tracheal resection) with endoscopic dilation [55]. Open reconstruction proved to be more cost-effective and exhibited higher quality-adjusted life year value compared with serial endoscopic dilations in select patients over 5- and 10-year time horizons [55]. The study commented that their findings should be most readily interpreted for patients who have long life expectancy, short dilation intervals, and few comorbid conditions as the opposite of these factors could change the cost-analysis conclusions.

Level of evidence	Conclusion
4	Open resection and reconstruction surgeries are more cost-effective than serial endoscopic dilations for select patients over a 5- and 10-year horizon [55]

More studies are needed in the future to better delineate the benefit of open surgical approaches over other management options in the management of laryngotracheal stenosis.

To date, the available literature does not have any randomized control trials comparing outcomes of endoscopic versus open surgical management of laryngotracheal stenosis. However, a large-scale, international, multi-institutional prospective cohort study (NoAAC PR-02 Study; ClinicalTrials.gov Identifier: NCT02481817; Start date: August 2015) is currently being conducted by the North American Airway Collaborative in order to study treatment outcomes in idiopathic subglottic stenosis compared between endoscopic dilations, endoscopic resections, and tracheal resections. With over 40 participating institutions and over 1000 participants anticipated, the study is estimated to conclude in October 2020. Primary outcome measures include time to recurrent procedure and need for tracheostomy over a follow-up time of 3 years. Secondary outcome measures focus on patient reported quality-of-life assessments in vocalizing, breathing, swallowing, and disease anxiety and burden.

Level of evidence	Conclusion
2	The North American Airway Collaborative is currently conducting a prospective, cohort study to examine treatment outcomes in idiopathic subglottic stenosis comparing different surgical treatment modalities; results expected after October 2020

Tracheostomy

Tracheostomy is another option which may be considered for patients with unrelenting stenosis and compromised airway. As a surgical procedure involving an incision of the anterior neck through the trachea, it is used in to help relieve acute airway distress or to secure the airway for subsequent endoscopic or surgical intervention. Temporary tracheostomy is performed with an end goal of decannulation whereas permanent tracheostomy commonly results from failure of surgical management to correct the stenosis. In one of the largest published care series to date on adult laryngotracheal stenosis, studying 340 patients, those with long stenosis, severe stenosis, or stenosis involving multiple subsites had a higher incidence of undergoing tracheostomy [2]. However, when stratified by etiology, this trend was most pronounced in iatrogenic laryngotracheal stenosis and not observed in patients who suffered from idiopathic laryngotracheal stenosis, suggesting that mechanism of injury is highly influential in rates of tracheostomy dependence [2].

Level of evidence	Conclusion
4	Patients with laryngotracheal stenosis secondary to non-idiopathic etiologies who have long, severe, or multisite stenosis have a higher incidence of tracheostomy [2]

Nonsurgical Management

Topical and Oral Adjuvant Therapies

Due to the contribution of inflammation and aberrant wound-healing to the pathophysiology of laryngotracheal stenosis, several adjuvant nonsurgical treatments are available to target these processes [56]. The efficacies of different topical and oral therapeutic pharmacologics are discussed here. Perhaps the most investigated adjuvant therapy in the management of laryngotracheal stenosis is mitomycin C. As an alkylating agent produced by the bacterium *Streptomyces caespitosus*, mitomycin C has been shown to strongly inhibit fibroblastic proliferation when applied topically [56]. Since its introduction as an adjuvant treatment option after surgery for airway stenosis in 1998, mitomycin C has become commonly accepted and routinely used in practice [57]. Most publications surrounding this topic in current literature are retrospective case-series studies that demonstrate improved outcomes, but there is still a paucity of high-level evidence-based studies to investigate its true efficacy [56, 58–60].

In Perepelitsyn et al., outcomes measured by success (improvement in airway symptoms or no need for further operative intervention) of endoscopic treatment of laryngotracheal stenosis were compared between three different groups: CO_2 laser only, laser with intralesional steroid injection, and laser with topical mitomycin C application [58]. It was reported that endoscopic intervention was associated with a statistically significant increase in treatment success from <20% to 75% when topical mitomycin C (0.04 mg/mL) was added as adjuvant therapy [58]. Furthermore, another study reviewing 71 patient charts demonstrated that the adjuvant use of mitomycin C lengthened the symptom-free period between endoscopic CO_2 laser procedures from 178 days without mitomycin C to 360 days ($p = 0.015$) [59].

Level of evidence	Conclusion
4	According to some retrospective studies, topical mitomycin C appears to be an effective adjuvant treatment in the endoscopic management of laryngotracheal stenosis [58, 59]

However, recent literature review reveals a less promising perspective on the efficacy of mitomycin C. In Wang et al., it was found on univariate analysis that mitomycin C was an independent risk factor for anastomotic complications and recurrence of stenosis after a laryngotracheal resection and the authors recommended against its use [50]. Smith et al. carried out a randomized, prospective, double-blinded trial that examined the relative benefit of multiple applications of mitomycin C versus only one [61]. Patients underwent three separate endoscopic dilations spaced 3–4 weeks and then 8–10 weeks apart, and they were randomized into two groups: one received topical mitomycin C (0.5 mg/mL) in the first two surgeries, and the other received mitomycin C in the first, and placebo in the second. They found that two applications of topical mitomycin C reduced the restenosis rate for 2–3 years after treatment when compared with only a single application. However, the 5-year relapse rate was found to be the same between both groups (69% versus 70%, respectively), suggesting that mitomycin C may postpone, but not prevent, the recurrence of symptomatic stenosis for patients [61]. While the comparison in this study was focused on differences in number of applications of mitomycin C, a prospective, randomized, double-blind, placebo-controlled study recently published by Yung et al. was the first study to compare the efficacy of topical mitomycin C (0.4 mg/mL) following endoscopic surgery compared to a placebo-controlled group in the treatment of laryngotracheal stenosis patients [62]. While limited by a small number of patients, the trial reported data from preliminary enrollment of 15 patients and demonstrated no statistically significant difference in average interval between surgical treatments, magnitude in peak inspiratory flow improvement, magnitude of symptom improvement, or duration of symptom improvement between the two groups ($p = 0.95$, 0.64, 0.73, 0.52, respectively) [62].

Level of evidence	Conclusion
2	Adjuvant use of topical mitomycin C has no additional benefit in the endoscopic surgical management of laryngotracheal stenosis [62]

Because of the heterogeneity in findings within the literature and scarcity of high-level evidence-based studies regarding this topic, further investigations are needed to better elucidate the definitive utility of mitomycin C in the treatment of laryngotracheal stenosis.

Another emerging approach is the use of immunomodulating agents, of which low-dose oral methotrexate has recently been studied. One retrospective case series study examined the use of methotrexate as an adjuvant therapy to surgical management for laryngotracheal stenosis and found that once-weekly treatment of 15 or 20 mg oral methotrexate increased the surgery-free interval by 251 days (95% CI, 193–309 days) after initiation [63].

Level of evidence	Conclusion
4	Low-dose adjunct oral methotrexate therapy initiation significantly increases the surgery-free interval for laryngotracheal stenosis patients [63]

Although generally well-tolerated among the cohort of ten patients, there were a few adverse effects reported in which two patients experienced mild hair thinning and onychomycosis and one patient developed a herpes zoster infection. More studies are necessary to determine if this clinical efficacy can be replicated and applied to large-scale LTS patient populations.

While acid reflux has been studied for years as a comorbidity and likely contributor to the pathophysiology behind adult laryngotracheal stenosis, the exact extent is not clear [50, 60, 64]. The use of oral adjuvant antigastroesophageal reflux therapy has not been studied extensively in controlled, prospective studies for laryngotracheal stenosis, but some initial reports indicate successful outcomes such as symptomatic improvement with the use of anti-reflux medications [60, 65].

As anti-inflammatory agents, steroids are known to mitigate macrophage response and fibroblast proliferation, which makes them useful in managing airway inflammation [1, 60]. The highest-level evidence for oral steroid use with specific application to laryngotracheal stenosis is a randomized, double-blind, placebo-controlled clinical trial that failed to demonstrate efficacy when given as low-dose systemic therapy following dilation of postintubation stenosis [66]. In this study, a total of 105 patients were randomized (50 steroids, 55 placebo), and patients receiving prednisolone 15 mg daily after surgery had no significant differences in their surgery-free intervals or number of airway operations ($p = 0.115$, 0.102, respectively). However, comparing the patients who eventually required airway resection (28/50 steroids, 40/44 placebo), there was a statistically significant, small decrease in the required airway resection length in the steroid group (5.3 mm decrease, $p = 0.044$).

Level of evidence	Conclusion
1	Low-dose systemic steroids have no effect on surgery-free interval or number of dilations, but they can potentially reduce the amount of resected trachea for patients who ultimately undergo surgical resection [66]

Inhaled Corticosteroids

In theory, administering steroids via inhalation is an attractive option for patients with laryngotracheal stenosis. The medication is not given systemically, which limits side effects and allows for better tolerance of long-term use. Furthermore, the medication is directly applied to the disease process through the airway rather than via the circulatory system. However, these medications are generally better suited for deposition in the alveoli and small airways, as estimates of the percent deposited dose for inhaled medications in large airways are only approximately 20–33% [67]. While studies specific to inhaled corticosteroid use in laryngotracheal stenosis patients are scarce, one case study on a patient in acute airway distress secondary to postintubation tracheal stenosis reported symptomatic improvement within days, supported by objective improvements in expiratory and inspiratory flow after

5 days of inhaled treatment (beclomethasone aerosol 0.2 mg every 6 hours) [68]. Another study by Yokoi et al. demonstrated efficacy of inhaled budesonide (0.25 mg twice daily) for the treatment of postoperative tracheal granulation tissue in patients with congenital tracheal stenosis by way of significantly reducing required stenting procedures in patients with inhaled treatment [69].

Level of evidence	Conclusion
4	Inhaled budesonide can be effective for treatment of postoperative granulation tissue in patients with congenital laryngotracheal stenosis [69]

More research is needed to determine if inhaled corticosteroids have superiority to placebo in long-term disease control.

Intralesional Steroid Injections

Steroid injections for the treatment of laryngotracheal stenosis involve the direct injection of corticosteroids into the scarred segment to both target local inflammation and cause local collagen remodeling and atrophy, as seen in cutaneous keloid treatment. Commonly, intralesional injections are done with endoscopic dilations in the operating room to reduce inflammation triggered by the procedure itself [60]. Because patients often require serial endoscopic dilations, there have been numerous retrospective investigations conducted over the years that demonstrate some efficacy of intralesional steroid injections in the treatment of laryngotracheal stenosis [70–73]. However, these studies are limited by small patient numbers as well as by variable, nonstandard outcome measures. Although historically most studied in Wegener's granulomatosis (WG) patients with laryngotracheal stenosis due to the prominent inflammatory pathophysiology, studies have expanded to include non-WG. In Hoffman et al., 21 patients with WG-related laryngotracheal stenosis were injected intraoperatively with methylprednisolone acetate (1 mL of 40 mg/mL) into the stenotic area. Of the six patients with prior tracheostomies, four were able to be decannulated after initiating intralesional injections [73]. Likewise, in a study by Wolter et al., 12 patients (8 WG, 4 non-WG) received intralesional steroid injections of triamcinolone (1 mL of 40 mg/mL) and the only patient with a previous tracheostomy was able to be successfully decannulated [72]. No patients required new tracheostomies in either study.

Level of evidence	Conclusion
4	Intralesional steroid injections with endoscopic dilation can be an effective strategy to treat laryngotracheal stenosis, with associations like decannulation in patients with prior tracheostomies and no new tracheostomies [72, 73]

Given the existing literature surrounding intralesional steroid injection efficacy in the operating room setting, there has been an interest in the applicability of this intervention in the office setting. In the last few years, this concept has been explored with the development of serial intralesional steroid injections (SILSI). In Franco et al., objective airway improvement was measured by spirometry for 13 idiopathic subglottic stenosis patients (6 exclusively SILSI, 7 endoscopic dilation followed by SILSI); both groups demonstrated statistically significant improvements of approximately 20–25% of percent peak expiratory flow [74].

In another retrospective study by Hoffman et al., it was shown that average percent stenosis significantly decreased for patients undergoing serial injections and of 17 patients with idiopathic subglottic stenosis who had undergone at least three injections, 14 did not need to return to the operating room since the first injection [75]. Patients also subjectively found the steroid injections tolerable, rating the average pain score as 2.3/10 [75].

Furthermore, studies indicated that in patients undergoing repeated endoscopic dilations for LTS of multiple etiologies, the surgery-free interval increased significantly after the initiation of SILSI [76, 77]. In Bertelsen et al., the surgery-free interval improved from 10.1 to 22.6 months (mean difference, 12.5 months; 95% CI, −2.1 to 27.2 months), with 50% of patients with prior tracheostomies able to achieve decannulation [76]. These results were corroborated by a recently published study by Pan et al., in which the surgery-free interval was statistically significantly longer after initiation of office-based steroid injections (17.9 versus 9.5 months, respectively; $p = 0.0041$), with 10 out of 13 patients not requiring repeat endoscopic dilation at an average of 1.7 years follow-up [77]. No adverse events or complications were reported in either study.

Although the results from initial retrospective studies are promising, they point to the need for further prospective studies to be implemented comparing aspects such as efficacy, tolerance, cost, among others, with current procedural methods before this office-based modality can become mainstay for laryngotracheal stenosis treatment.

Level of evidence	Conclusion
4	Serial in-office intralesional steroid injections (SILSI) increase the surgery-free interval for laryngotracheal patients treated with serial endoscopic dilations. They are well-tolerated, with low pain scores. Patients treated exclusively with SILSI can see improvement in airway caliber to the same extent as those treated with endoscopic dilations followed by in-office SILSI [74–77]

Conclusion

Laryngotracheal stenosis is a rare, complex condition characterized by multifactorial etiologies and high recurrence rates. Despite various options for treatment, patients and providers often experience significant physiologic, psychosocial, and economic burdens when managing this disease. However, promising surgical and nonsurgical therapeutic approaches have been shown to have efficacy with positive outcomes. Endoscopic dilation and laryngotracheal resection may prove beneficial to manage airway compromise, and when combined with adjuvant nonsurgical therapy can greatly improve or resolve interval symptoms. Further studies at higher levels of evidence are required to establish clear benefits and provide structure for standardized management.

References

1. Rosow DE, Barbarite E. Review of adult laryngotracheal stenosis: pathogenesis, management, and outcomes. Curr Opin Otolaryngol Head Neck Surg. 2016;24(6):489–93.
2. Gelbard A, Francis DO, Sandulache VC, et al. Causes and consequences of adult laryngotracheal stenosis. Laryngoscope. 2015;125(5):1137–43.
3. Kocdor P, Siegel ER, Suen JY, et al. Comorbidities and factors associated with endoscopic surgical outcomes in adult laryngotracheal stenosis. Eur Arch Otorhinolaryngol. 2016;273(2):419–24.
4. Nouraei SA, Nouraei SM, Patel A, et al. Diagnosis of laryngotracheal stenosis from routine pulmonary physiology using the expiratory disproportion index. Laryngoscope. 2013;123(12):3099–104.
5. De Benedictis FM, de Benedictis D, Mirabile L, et al. Ground zero: not asthma at all. Pediatr Allergy Immunol. 2015;26:490–6.
6. Gnagi SH, Howard BE, Anderson C, et al. Idiopathic subglottic and & tracheal stenosis: a survey of the patient experience. Ann Otol Rhinol Laryngol. 2015;124:734–9.
7. Stauffer JL, Olson DE, Petty TL. Complications and consequences of endotracheal intubation and tracheotomy. A prospective study of 150 critically ill adult patients. Am J Med. 1981;70:65–76.
8. Seegobin RD, van Hasselt GL. Endotracheal cuff pressure and tracheal mucosal blood flow: endoscopic study of effects of four large volume cuffs. Br Med J (Clin Res Ed). 1984;288:965–8.
9. Halum SL, Ting JY, Plowman EK, et al. A multiinstitutional analysis of tracheotomy complications. Laryngoscope. 2012;122:38–45.
10. Lahav Y, Shoffel-Havakuk H, Halperin D. Acquired glottic stenosis-the ongoing challenge: a review of etiology, pathogenesis, and surgical management. J Voice. 2015;29(5):646.e1–646.e10.
11. Gadkaree SK, Pandian V, Best S, Motz KM, et al. Laryngotracheal stenosis: risk factors for tracheostomy dependence and dilation interval. Otolaryngol Head Neck Surg. 2017;156(2):321–8.
12. Almouhawis HA, Leao JC, Fedele S, et al. Wegener's granulomatosis: a review of clinical features and an update in diagnosis and treatment. J Oral Pathol Med. 2013;42(7):507–16.

13. Dablanca M, Maeso A, Méndez DD, et al. Laryngotracheal stenosis of autoimmune aetiology. Acta Otorrinolaringol Esp. 2017;68(1):38–42.

14. Gelbard A, Katsantonis NG, Mizuta M, et al. Idiopathic subglottic stenosis is associated with activation of the inflammatory IL-17A/IL-23 axis. Laryngoscope. 2016;126(11):E356–61.

15. Koufman JA. The otolaryngologic manifestations of gastroesophageal reflux disease (GERD): a clinical investigation of 225 patients using ambulatory 24-hour pH monitoring and an experimental investigation of the role of acid and pepsin in the development of laryngeal injury. Laryngoscope. 1991;101:1–78.

16. Maronian NC, Azadeh H, Waugh P, et al. Association of laryngopharyngeal reflux disease and subglottic stenosis. Ann Otol Rhinol Laryngol. 2001;110:606–11.

17. Aldhahrani A, Powell J, Ladak S, et al. The potential role of bile acids in acquired Laryngotracheal stenosis. Laryngoscope. 2018;128(9):2029–33.

18. McCann AJ, Samuels TL, Blumin JH, et al. The role of pepsin in epithelia-mesenchymal transition in idiopathic subglottic stenosis. Laryngoscope. 2020;130(1):154–8.

19. Vanaudenaerde BM, De Vleeschauwer SI, Vos R, et al. The role of the IL23/IL17 axis in bronchiolitis obliterans syndrome after lung transplantation. Am J Transplant. 2008;8(9):1911–20.

20. Morrison RJ, Katsantonis NG, Motz KM, et al. Pathologic fibroblasts in idiopathic subglottic stenosis amplify local inflammatory signals. Otolaryngol Head Neck Surg. 2019;160(1):107–15.

21. Nicolli EA, Ghosh A, Haft S, et al. IL-1 receptor antagonist inhibits early granulation formation. Ann Otol Rhinol Laryngol. 2016;125(4):284–9.

22. Hillel AT, Tang SS, Carlos C, et al. Laryngotracheal microbiota in adult laryngotracheal stenosis. mSphere. 2019;4(3):e00211–9.

23. Costantino CL, Mathisen DJ. Idiopathic laryngotracheal stenosis. J Thorac Dis. 2016;8(Suppl 2):S204–9.

24. Monnier P, Dikkers FG, Eckel H, et al. Preoperative assessment and classification of benign laryngotracheal stenosis: a consensus paper of the European Laryngological Society. Eur Arch Otorhinolaryngol. 2015;272:2885–96.

25. Myer CM 3rd, O'Connor DM, Cotton RT. Proposed grading system for subglottic stenosis based on endotracheal tube sizes. Ann Otol Rhinol Laryngol. 1994;103:319–23.

26. Hall SR, Allen CT, Merati AL, et al. Evaluating the utility of serological testing in laryngotracheal stenosis. Laryngoscope. 2017;127(6):1408–12.

27. Ossoff RH, Sisson GA, Duncavage JA, et al. Endoscopic laser arytenoidectomy for the treatment of bilateral vocal cord paralysis. Laryngoscope. 1984;94(10):1293–7.

28. Yilmaz T. Endoscopic partial arytenoidectomy for bilateral vocal fold paralysis: medially based mucosal flap technique. J Voice. 2019;33(5):751–8. pii: S0892-1997(18)30100-0.

29. Dedo HH, Sooy CD. Endoscopic laser repair of posterior glottic, subglottic and tracheal stenosis by division or micro-trapdoor flap. Laryngoscope. 1984;94(4):445–50.

30. Dennis DP, Kashima H. Carbon dioxide laser posterior cordectomy for treatment of bilateral vocal cord paralysis. Ann Otol Rhinol Laryngol. 1989;98(12 Pt 1):930–4.

31. Riffat F, Palme CE, Veivers D. Endoscopic treatment of glottic stenosis: a report on the safety and efficacy of CO2 laser. J Laryngol Otol. 2011;126(5):503–5.

32. Leventhal DD, Krebs E, Rosen MR. Flexible laser bronchoscopy for subglottic stenosis in the awake patient. Arch Otolaryngol Head Neck Surg. 2009;135(5):467–71.

33. Ciccone AM, De Giacomo T, Venuta F, et al. Operative and non-operative treatment of benign subglottic laryngotracheal stenosis. Eur J Cardiothorac Surg. 2004;26(4):818–22.

34. Mehta AC, Lee FY, Cordasco EM, et al. Concentric tracheal and subglottic stenosis. Management using the Nd-YAG laser for mucosal sparing followed by gentle dilatation. Chest. 1993;104(3):673–7.

35. Anand VK, Galantich PT. Advantages of endoscopic laser arytenoidectomy using yag laser scalpel. J Voice. 1990;4(2):165–8.

36. Hu Y, Cheng L, Liu B, et al. The assistance of coblation in arytenoidectomy for vocal cord paralysis. Acta Otolaryngol. 2019;139(1):90–3.

37. Monnier P, George M, Monod ML, et al. The role of the CO2 laser in the management of laryngotracheal stenosis: a survey of 100 cases. Eur Arch Otorhinolaryngol. 2005;262(8):602–8.

38. Herrington HC, Weber SM, Andersen PE. Modern management of laryngotracheal stenosis. Laryngoscope. 2006;116(9):1553–7.

39. Hseu AF, Benninger MS, Haffey TM, et al. Subglottic stenosis: a ten-year review of treatment outcomes. Laryngoscope. 2014;124(3):736–41.

40. Maresh A, Preciado DA, O'Connell AP, et al. A comparative analysis of open surgery vs endoscopic balloon dilation for pediatric subglottic stenosis. JAMA Otolaryngol Head Neck Surg. 2014;140(10):901–5.

41. Lang M, Brietzke SE. A systematic review and meta-analysis of endoscopic balloon dilation of pediatric subglottic stenosis. Otolaryngol Head Neck Surg. 2013;150(2):174–9.

42. Sinacori JT, Taliercio SJ, Duong E, et al. Modalities of treatment for laryngotracheal stenosis: the EVMS experience. Laryngoscope. 2013;123(12):3131–6.

43. Hillel AT, Karatayli-Ozgursoy S, Benke JR, et al. Voice quality in laryngotracheal stenosis: impact of dilation and level of stenosis. Ann Otol Rhinol Laryngol. 2015;124(5):413–8.

44. Hoffman MR, Brand WT, Dailey SH. Effects of balloon dilation for idiopathic Laryngotracheal stenosis on voice production. Ann Otol Rhinol Laryngol. 2016 Jan;125(1):12–9.

45. Lewis S, Earley M, Rosenfeld R, et al. Systematic review for surgical treatment of adult and adolescent laryngotracheal stenosis. Laryngoscope. 2017;127(1):191–8.
46. Yamamoto K, Kojima F, Tomiyama K, et al. Meta-analysis of therapeutic procedures for acquired subglottic stenosis in adults. Ann Thorac Surg. 2011;91(6):1747–53.
47. Hsu YB, Damrose EJ. Safety of outpatient airway dilation for adult laryngotracheal stenosis. Ann Otol Rhinol Laryngol. 2015;124(6):452–7.
48. Valdez TA, Shapshay SM. Idiopathic subglottic stenosis revisited. Ann Otol Rhinol Laryngol. 2002;111(8):690–5.
49. Parker NP, Bandyopadhyay D, Misono S, et al. Endoscopic cold incision, balloon dilation, mitomycin C application, and steroid injection for adult laryngotracheal stenosis. Laryngoscope. 2013;123(1):220–5.
50. Wang H, Wright CD, Wain JC, et al. Idiopathic subglottic stenosis: factors affecting outcome after single-stage repair. Ann Thorac Surg. 2015;100(5):1804–11.
51. Auchincloss HG, Wright CD. Complications after tracheal resection and reconstruction: prevention and treatment. J Thorac Dis. 2016;8(Suppl 2):S160–7.
52. Wright CD, Grillo HC, Wain JC, et al. Anastomotic complications after tracheal resection: prognostic factors and management. J Thorac Cardiovasc Surg. 2004;128(5):731–9.
53. Clunie GM, Kinshuck AJ, Sandhu GS, et al. Voice and swallowing outcomes for adults undergoing reconstructive surgery for laryngotracheal stenosis. Curr Opin Otolaryngol Head Neck Surg. 2017;25(3):195–9.
54. Lennon CJ, Gelbard A, Bartow C, et al. Dysphagia following airway reconstruction in adults. JAMA Otolaryngol Head Neck Surg. 2016;142:20–4.
55. Yin LX, Padula WV, Gadkaree S, et al. Health care costs and cost-effectiveness in laryngotracheal stenosis. Otolaryngol Head Neck Surg. 2019;160(4):679–86.
56. Hirshoren N, Eliashar R. Wound-healing modulation in upper airway stenosis- myths and facts. Head Neck. 2009;31(1):111–26.
57. Ward RF, April MM. Mitomycin-C in the treatment of tracheal cicatrix after tracheal reconstruction. Int J Pediatr Otorhinolaryngol. 1998;44:221–6.
58. Perepelitsyn I, Shapshay SM. Endoscopic treatment of laryngeal and tracheal stenosis- has mitomycin C improved the outcome? Otolaryngol Head Neck Surg. 2004;131(1):16–20.
59. Reichert LK, Zhao AS, Galati LT, et al. The efficacy of mitomycin C in the treatment of laryngotracheal stenosis: results and experiences with a difficult disease entity. ORL J Otorhinolaryngol Relat Spec. 2015;77:351–8.
60. Maldonado F, Loiselle A, DePew ZS, et al. Idiopathic subglottic stenosis: an evolving therapeutic algorithm. Laryngoscope. 2014;124(2):498–503.
61. Smith ME, Elstad M. Mitomycin C and the endoscopic treatment of laryngotracheal stenosis: are two applications better than one? Laryngoscope. 2009;119(2):272–83.

62. Yung KC, Chang J, Courey MS. A randomized control trial of adjuvant mitomycin-c in endoscopic surgery for laryngotracheal stenosis. Laryngoscope. 2020;130(3):706–11.

63. Rosow DE, Ahmed J. Initial experience with low-dose methotrexate as an adjuvant treatment for rapidly recurrent nonvasculitic laryngotracheal stenosis. JAMA Otolaryngol Head Neck Surg. 2017;143(2):125–30.

64. Jindal JR, Milbrath MM, Shaker R, et al. Gastroesophageal reflux disease as a likely cause of "idiopathic" subglottic stenosis. Ann Otol Rhinol Laryngol. 1994;103(3):186–91.

65. Terra RM, de Medeiros IL, Minamoto H, et al. Idiopathic tracheal stenosis: successful outcome with antigastroesophageal reflux disease therapy. Ann Thorac Surg. 2008;85(4):1438–9.

66. Shadmehr MB, Abbasidezfouli A, Farzanegan R, et al. The role of systemic steroids in postintubation tracheal stenosis: a randomized clinical trial. Ann Thorac Surg. 2017;103(1):246–53.

67. Anderson M, Svartengren M, Camner P. Human tracheobronchial deposition and effect of a cholinergic aerosol inhaled by extremely slow inhalations. Exp Lung Res. 1999;25(4):335–52.

68. Braidy J, Breton G, Clement L. Effect of corticosteroids on postintubation tracheal stenosis. Thorax. 1989;44(9):753–5.

69. Yokoi A, Nakao M, Bitoh Y, et al. Treatment of postoperative tracheal granulation tissue with inhaled budesonide in congenital tracheal stenosis. J Pediatr Surg. 2014;49(2):293–5.

70. Gnanapragasam A. Intralesional steroids in conservative management of subglottic stenosis of the larynx. Int Surg. 1979;64:63–7.

71. Cobb WB, Sudderth JF. Intralesional steroids in laryngeal stenosis. Arch Otolaryngol. 1972;96:52–6.

72. Wolter NE, Ooi EH, Witterick IJ. Intralesional corticosteroid injection and dilatation provides effective management of subglottic stenosis in Wegener's granulomatosis. Laryngoscope. 2010;120(12):2452–5.

73. Hoffman GS, Thomas-Golbanov CK, Chan J, et al. Treatment of subglottic stenosis, due to Wegener's granulomatosis, with intralesional corticosteroids and dilation. J Rheumatol. 2003;30(5):1017–21.

74. Franco RA Jr, Husain I, Reder L, et al. Awake serial intralesional steroid injections without surgery as a novel treatment for idiopathic subglottic stenosis. Laryngoscope. 2018;128(3):610–7.

75. Hoffman MR, Coughlin AR, Dailey SH. Serial office-based steroid injections for treatment of idiopathic subglottic stenosis. Laryngoscope. 2017;127(11):2475–81.

76. Bertelsen C, Shoffel-Havakuk H, O'Dell K, et al. Serial in-office intralesional steroid injections in airway stenosis. JAMA Otolaryngol Head Neck Surg. 2018;144(3):203–10.

77. Pan DR, Rosow DE. Office-based corticosteroid injections as adjuvant therapy for subglottic stenosis. Laryngoscope Investig Otolaryngol. 2019;4:414.

Dysphagia

9

Angelina Schache and Ashli O'Rourke

Introduction

Dysphagia impacts approximately 1 in 25 adults in the United States, and this number continues to grow [1]. According to multiple reports, older adults are more likely to experience dysphagia [1–4]. Dysphagia can arise from a variety of causes, such as cerebral vascular accidents, head and neck cancer, neurologic diseases, rheumatoid disorders, and/or surgical interventions. Associated signs and symptoms of dysphagia can include coughing, choking, globus sensation, regurgitation, odynophagia, drooling, unexplained weight loss, nutritional deficiencies, and/or aspiration pneumonia [2, 5, 6].

There are many approaches to the evaluation and management of dysphagia. The last 10 years has seen an exponential rise in dysphagia-related publications but unfortunately, the majority of studies represent smaller sample sizes at single institutions. To better

A. Schache
Department of Otolaryngology - Head and Neck Surgery, University of Washington School of Medicine, Seattle, WA, USA

A. O'Rourke (✉)
Evelyn Trammell Institute for Voice & Swallowing, Department of Otolaryngology - Head and Neck Surgery, Medical University of South Carolina, Charleston, SC, USA
e-mail: aorourke@musc.edu

© Springer Nature Switzerland AG 2021   175
D. E. Rosow, C. M. Ivey (eds.), *Evidence-Based Laryngology*,
https://doi.org/10.1007/978-3-030-58494-8_9

understand the evidence that underpins best practices in dysphagia care, we conducted a literature search limited to the past 10 years. We included the search terms "dysphagia," "swallowing disorders," and "deglutition" and filtered the results by adult, English language, and human trials. We excluded esophageal dysphagia studies to focus on oropharyngeal issues. From these articles, we selected those with large cohorts (evidence level IIb), randomized control trials (RCTs) (evidence level Ib), systematic reviews (evidence level Ia – IIIa), and meta-analyses (evidence level Ia – IIIa) [7].

We will discuss pertinent topics within swallowing physiology, diagnosis, and treatment of swallowing disorders with reference to the available literature in hopes this chapter will be a useful reference for guiding treatment decisions.

Swallowing Physiology

Effective swallowing is crucial for maintaining adequate nutrition, hydration, and quality of life. Swallowing is a complex neuromuscular process involving more than 50 muscles and several cranial nerves [8]. Precise coordination is required to elicit the requisite volitional and reflexive activities that pass a bolus from the oral cavity to the esophagus. Impairments in swallowing can have devastating effects on a person's physical and mental health.

Normal swallowing function has both reflexive and voluntary components that change with growth and development. In the adult, pre-oral, oral, oropharyngeal, pharyngoesophageal, and esophageal phases have been defined for swallowing function. Swallow dysfunction may occur during any of these phases, and it is often multilevel in cases of neurologic and systemic disease. The following studies have value in understanding swallow mechanics and how they may be affected.

The Aging Swallow

As with other parts of the human body, the swallowing mechanism changes with age. A prospective population-based cohort study evaluated 47 "old-old" women aged 85–94 who reported no dysphagia and had no history of neurologic disease [9]. The subjects were challenged with the 3-ounce water test, which asks participants to drink 3 ounces (90 ml) of water without interruption. The investigators measured stoppage before finishing the entire amount, choking, coughing, throat clearing, and/or presence of a wet sounding voice. They found that 72% of participants (34/47) exhibited swallowing dysfunction on at least one of three challenges and 34% (16/47) had difficulty on all three challenges. Frailty did not correlate with swallowing dysfunction [9]. It should be noted that the 3-ounce water test is a screening examination, and confirmatory evaluation was not completed in this study. In addition, the consequences of dysphagia (e.g. pneumonia, weight loss) were not directly evaluated. This study, however, strengthens the argument that some swallowing dysfunction is expected in older individuals and clinicians should evaluate the safety of swallowing function and the actual effect of dysfunction prior to intervention.

Bolus Modification and Dysphagia

A paper published by the European Society of Swallowing Disorders examined the effect of bolus viscosity modifications in patients with oropharyngeal dysphagia [10]. Thirty-three articles were considered, including randomized controlled trials and systematic reviews. The group found that while the safety of swallowing (i.e. aspiration and penetration) improved with increasing viscosity, more viscous boluses also correlated with increased pharyngeal residue, decreased palatability, and increased risk of dehydration [10]. The group suggested that newer type thickening agents, other than xanthan gum and starch, are necessary to help with compliance. Additionally, they recommended that patients on thickened liquids be monitored for dehydration.

Leonard et al. evaluated the difference between starch- and gum-based thickeners in a prospective double-blinded clinical trial specifically evaluating the prevalence of penetration and aspiration. They found less aspiration with gum thickener versus thin liquids but there was no difference in aspiration between starch and gum or starch and thin liquids. Some have hypothesized that gum-based thickeners may be more stable than starch-based thickeners, as the latter are broken down by amylase present in the saliva. Leonard et al. propose that the difference between the two thickeners is likely related to other rheological properties such as shear and flow rate versus viscosity measurements alone [11].

Kaneoka et al. evaluated whether patients who aspirated thin liquids were at higher risk of developing pneumonia if they consumed only thickened liquids compared to patients who drank water between meals while using swallowing strategies. Their meta-analysis and systematic review of seven studies and 650 patients compared the effects of viscosity modification, thin water protocols, and postural adjustments. They found that patients who drank water with strategies between meals had a similar rate of pneumonia as those in the control condition. Additionally, they determined that the experimental group had better hydration and overall quality of life [12]. It is also crucial to mention that good oral care has a large impact on these results, as this is a large contributor to decreased pneumonia risk [13–16].

Other bolus properties besides viscosity may affect swallowing physiology. Michou et al. evaluated the effect of carbonation and temperature on swallowing reaction time in 39 normal younger adults (mean age 27.7 years). They found that carbonation resulted in more success during a challenge scenario where the subject was required to swallow at timed intervals. Cold water swallows had significantly shortened swallow latency during normal swallowing condition but no other differences were found in fast swallows or timed challenge swallowing conditions [17]. Another interesting double-blinded, randomized study showed that a 1 mM solution of piperine (the pungent ingredient in black pepper) mixed in a nectar bolus reduced penetration and aspiration scores in severely dysphagic adults [18]. It is hypothesized that neurostimulation may be helpful to improve swallowing in patients.

Nasogastric Catheters and Dysphagia

Another common physiologic question is whether the presence of a catheter or nasogastric tube affects swallowing in a clinically meaningful way. Huggins et al. had previously shown no differences in airway protection or bolus clearance in young normal volunteers based on nasogastric tube presence [19]. However, in an equally small ($n = 9$) randomized controlled crossover trial, Pryor et al. showed that in older nondysphagic adults, nasogastric tubes were associated with increased penetration and aspiration in some swallowing conditions (serial liquid and puree swallows) as well as increased residue (puree) [20]. The difference in results between these two studies may be confounded by age-related swallowing differences and small sample sizes, so results should be interpreted with caution.

Local Anesthesia Effects on Swallowing Mechanics

The effect of local anesthesia on the physiology of swallowing has been debated for many years. This mainly has relevance to flexible endoscopic evaluation of swallowing (FEES), sensory testing, and pharyngeal manometric testing. Odea et al. performed a single (participant) blinded crossover study with 17 dysphagic patients aged 45–85 years (mean age 62 years). Patients were administered 0.2 ml of 4% lidocaine with a decongestant (experimental group) versus decongestant only in a control group. The authors found no difference between penetration, aspiration, or residue in the experimental versus control condition during FEES but did note that pain during scope insertion and average pain scores were lower in the anesthetized condition [21]. These results were similar to a cross over study by Kamarunas, where no clinically significant differences in swallowing physiology or sensory testing were found between anesthetized versus control groups [22]. However Fife et al. found that while there was less discomfort and similar penetration aspiration scale scores, that a higher score was 33% more likely when anesthesia was used [23].

In a double-blinded study in normal individuals, Hernandez et al. evaluated changes in manometric pressures during swallowing in anesthetized versus nonanesthetized conditions. The experimental group had application of 0.4 ml of 2% viscous lidocaine on a cotton tip applicator and had statistically significant reduction in pharyngeal pressures [24]. However, the differences were small and given the known variability of manometric measures, the clinical relevance of the reduction remains unclear.

Level of evidence	Conclusion
2	Cold temperature water may improve swallow initiation times [17]
3	Increased viscosity of liquids decreases rate of penetration or aspiration but increases pharyngeal residue, decreases palatability, and may increase risk of dehydration [10]
2	Judicious use of anesthesia, that is limited as much as possible to the nasal cavity, has little effect on swallowing physiology and can improve patient tolerance and comfort for invasive instrumental examinations [21–23]

Dysphagia Diagnostics

Screening

It is imperative to determine which patients in an at-risk population may have swallowing difficulty in order to further elucidate their problem and offer effective treatment. Screening tools have been developed in order to identify the patients most likely to be affected. Kertscher et al. assessed the quality and utility of the available dysphagia screening tools for patients in a systematic review with focus on sensitivity, specificity, and reliability data. The Toronto Bedside Swallowing Screening and the 3oz. Water Swallowing Test were found to have high sensitivity, but only moderate specificity [25]. In 2017, the Gugging Swallowing

Screen was studied by Warnecke et al. in a prospective, double-blinded fashion, and was also found to have high sensitivity but modest specificity [26]. These assessments can be provided bedside by a health practitioner and are helpful in pinpointing patients with high risk, but given their low specificity, should not be thought to completely rule out possibility of dysphagia.

Level of evidence	Conclusion
2	Swallowing screening can assist in identification of at-risk individuals, but specificity is low, so negative testing may be suspect [25, 26]

Diagnostic Testing

Most diagnostic testings combine a modality to visualize the upper aerodigestive system with standardized assessment tools to evaluate swallowing function. The most commonly used assessment tool is the Penetration-Aspiration Scale (PAS). This specifically measures the depth of penetration of matter into the airway during a swallow in order to stratify aspiration potential. PAS was shown in a cohort study to differentiate normal subjects from both stroke patients and head and neck cancer patients [27]. This information, along with motor assessment and clinical judgment, allows the swallowing therapist or physician to assess the severity of dysphagia and suggest interventions that may improve swallowing and decrease potential for aspiration. Use of the PAS allows for standardized communication and evaluation of an otherwise very complicated and nuanced disorder, and its clinical utility in multiple modalities has been evaluated [28].

Swallowing fluoroscopy is considered the gold standard for diagnosis of dysphagia, and much attention has been placed on standardization of this test. This test can be ordered as a video swallowing evaluation (VSE, VSS) or a modified barium esophagram (MBS). It necessitates radiation and specific upright positioning in order to fully evaluate the oropharyngeal, nasopharyngeal, and pharyngoesophageal regions during swallow. It is very helpful for assessment of aspiration, as the column of contrast material can be visualized either penetrating or entering the glottis and upper airway during testing. While this test can be performed easily in most hospitals, a 2013 systemic review concluded that, although intra-rater reliability was high, methodology in test performance varied and interrater reliability was low. Overall reliability could be improved with applied bolus consistency, pretraining of raters, and consistency in measurement criteria [29].

FEES with or without sensory testing has many benefits that argue for its role as gold standard testing in dysphagia. Endoscopy is performed during swallowing maneuvers to get direct assessment of muscular propulsion of the bolus and any pooling, penetration, or aspiration of oropharyngeal contents. This study can be done at the bedside or in the clinic and does not necessitate radiation exposure or explicit positioning in order to obtain data, making it very popular for pediatric evaluation of dysphagia. There is approximately 0.5 s during the swallow when the upper airway soft tissue blocks visualization and limits the capability of FEES to evaluate direct penetration and aspiration. Nonetheless, prospective studies have shown high interrater reliability in assessment of swallow dysfunction [30].

Both fluoroscopy and FEES have important roles in the diagnosis of dysphagia, and the data observed may be complementary. They can be used diagnostically and for evaluation of intervention throughout swallowing therapy. One prospective study directly comparing these modalities showed that, while both were useful for assessing dysphagia, there were significant differences in scoring of PAS (higher scores noted on VSS), detection of aspiration (more caught on VSS), and extent of pooled residue (larger on FEES) [31].

Studies have looked at other diagnostic modalities that may be helpful to evaluate swallowing issues. These include, but are not limited to high-resolution manometry, pressure flow analysis (PFA), functional luminal imaging probe (FLIP), and accelerometry. These are mentioned in order to educate the reader about other examinations that may be available in certain centers, but that are not yet mainstream for basic diagnostic purposes [32].

Level of evidence	Conclusion
3	PAS can be effectively used to assess penetration and aspiration using a number of imaging modalities [27]
2/3	Fluoroscopic imaging techniques are gold-standard for assessment of aspiration and dysphagia, but need consistent measurement indices and bolus texture [29]
2	FEES is an easy and direct way to obtain reliable data concerning dysphagia but may miss aspiration events [31]

Dysphagia Treatment

A primary concern for individuals with dysphagia includes identifying the intervention needed to improve swallowing function. In planning a treatment, it is crucial to have detailed knowledge of the patient's medical status, previous or current treatments, and most importantly, have a clear vision of the patient's goals. In terms of selecting a treatment, this should be based on the best available current evidence from published literature.

In 2019 Bath et al. compared 41 randomized controlled trials to determine the overall efficacy of swallowing therapy and the types of interventions that were completed [33]. Interventions included behavioral interventions, drug therapies, acupuncture, neuromuscular stimulation, physical stimulation, transcranial direct stimulation, transcranial magnetic stimulation, and pharyngeal electrical stimulation. The conclusion showed that overall, swallowing therapy reduced the length of inpatient hospitalization, improved swallowing ability, and decreased the risk of pneumonia. As there were many different interventions completed, it is not clear which treatment was most effective.

Traditional Swallowing Therapy

Park et al. studied 22 patients following stroke and provided them with either conventional dysphagia therapy or chin tuck against resistance (CTAR) using a CTAR device [34]. They concluded that the CTAR group showed greater improvement in oral cavity, pyriform and vallecular residue, laryngeal elevation, and epiglottic inversion when compared with the patients in the control group.

Chen et al. completed a randomized controlled study evaluating whether tracheal traction exercises prior to ACDF surgery reduced the incidence of postoperative dysphagia [35]. Tracheal traction exercises involve manual manipulation of the thyroid cartilage from side to side which aims to increase the compliance of the cricopharyngeus and reduce the pressure required by retraction to maintain an adequate operative field. This study showed that patients who completed tracheal traction exercises prior to their surgery had a significantly lower incidence of dysphagia 1–3 weeks after their surgery [35]. However, there was no significant difference between the treatment and control groups at 6 weeks, 3 months, or 6 months postoperatively.

Moon et al. were interested in determining if tongue pressure strength and accuracy training (TPSAT), combined with traditional dysphagia therapy, would result in better outcomes for stroke survivors [36]. The Iowa Oral Performance Instrument (IOPI) device was used to measure anterior and posterior tongue pressures pre- and posttreatment. The experimental group received TPSAT and traditional dysphagia therapy, whereas the control group only received dysphagia therapy. The results indicated a reduced incidence of dysphagia and better quality of life outcomes for the patients who received both interventions compared with dysphagia therapy alone.

Fujimaki et al. examined whether glottic closure exercises could decrease the incidence of aspiration. They randomized 408 patients with glottic insufficiency due to vocal atrophy to vocal exercises ($N = 199$) versus education alone ($N = 209$). The outcome measure was development of clinical pneumonia with a 6-month endpoint. They found that the maximum phonation time was significantly increased in the experimental group ($p = 0.001$). Hospitalization for pneumonia was also significantly different between with the groups, with two patients in the exercise group developing pneumonia versus 18 in the control group ($p = 0.001$) [37]. Potential drawbacks of this study included no assessment of the pretreatment aspiration risk of the patients, and exclusion of patients who chose surgery from randomization.

Terre et al. performed a randomized alternating crossover study evaluating the effects of a chin tuck during swallowing in 47 neurogenic dysphagia patients versus 25 normal controls. The investigators found that the chin tuck maneuver decreased aspiration in 55% of patients in the experimental group and did not increase incidence of aspiration in the control group. The 45% of patients who continued to aspirate while utilizing a chin tuck had more delayed pharyngeal initiation, pharyngeal residue, and cricopharyngeal dysfunction when compared with the patients in whom the chin tuck alleviated aspiration. Viscosity had no effect on the efficacy of the chin tuck [38].

Level of evidence	Conclusion
1	The use of a therapeutic device for tongue strengthening exercises in combination with traditional dysphagia therapy improves patient outcomes [36]
2	Vocal exercises for glottic insufficiency, resulting from vocal cord atrophy, may increase airway protection and decrease the risk of developing pneumonia [37]
1	The implementation of a chin tuck in dysphagic patients can decrease the risk of aspiration as compared with controls (however, this strategy is not always effective in prevention of aspiration) [38]

Transcutaneous Neuromuscular Electrical Stimulation

A more novel approach to swallowing rehabilitation is the use of transcutaneous neuromuscular electrical stimulation (NMES). This practice is often used in rehabilitation facilities to increase muscle size, range of motion, endurance, and muscle strength

[39]. A randomized controlled trial of 16 healthy subjects utilized NMES as an adjunct to effortful swallowing exercises while a control group received sub-therapeutic electrical stimulation [40]. NMES increased hyoid elevation in this population but the effect faded within 2 weeks following treatment.

Chen et al. completed a meta-analysis of eight randomized and quasi-randomized controlled trials that utilized NMES to treat post-stroke dysphagia. The researchers evaluated the effects of three conditions: (1) NMES combined with traditional swallowing therapy, (2) NMES alone, and (3) traditional swallowing therapy alone. Overall, the conclusion was that neuromuscular electrical stimulation, in combination with dysphagia therapy, was more effective in the short term than swallow therapy alone in post-stroke patients. There was not sufficient evidence to determine if NMES alone was superior to swallowing therapy alone [41]. This study was limited by heterogeneity of the patient population and high variability of outcome measures.

Tan et al. also performed a meta-analysis assessing the efficacy of NMES versus "traditional" swallowing therapy. Seven studies were included in the meta-analysis with 291 patients (175 NMES and 116 receiving traditional therapy). The quality of included studies was high with three randomized controlled studies and four clinical controlled trials. Interestingly, the meta-analysis revealed that NMES was more effective than traditional therapy in nonstroke etiologies (e.g. Parkinson's disease or head and neck cancer) but in the stroke group subset, there was no difference between the treatment methods [42]. This finding was similar to those by other authors [41, 43].

Ortega et al. evaluated the effects of electrical (NMES) versus chemical stimulation on the rehabilitation of swallowing. The chemical intervention used was a transient receptor potential vanillin 1 agonist. They found that chronic sensory stimulation strategies reduced the prevalence of oropharyngeal dysphagia and may promote recovery of impaired swallowing function [44]. Similarly Konecny et al. observed the effects of electrically stimulating the hyoid muscles of post-stroke patients with dysphagia for 20 minutes per day in addition to orofacial rehabilitation (OFR) [45]. They found statistically significant changes in the duration of the oropharyngeal transit times of the patients who completed both OFR and electrical stimulation versus patients in the control group who received only OFR. Lim et al. discovered that the combination of electrical stimulation and thermal tactile stimulation resulted in better outcomes than thermal tactile stimulation alone [46].

Level of evidence	Conclusion
1	Neuromuscular electrical stimulation, when combined with other treatment modalities, may improve swallowing outcomes [40–46]

Transcranial Stimulation

Pisegna et al. performed a meta-analysis evaluating the effects of transcranial direct current stimulation (tDCS) and repetitive transcranial magnetic stimulation (rTMS) on post-stroke dysphagia patients. Eight randomized trials, with a total of 146 patients, were included and factors such as stimulation of the affected versus unaffected hemisphere, stimulation duration, stimulation type, electric field orientation, and long-term follow up effects were analyzed. It was found that noninvasive brain stimulation increased the excitability of the corticobulbar projections and in turn, increased neuroplasticity and positively affected the cortical swallowing network [47]. Though larger randomized-controlled trials are necessary to further determine the outcome of noninvasive brain stimulation on post-stroke dysphagia patients, this study concluded that there is evidence of efficacy of stimulating the unaffected hemisphere rather than the affected one.

Level of evidence	Conclusion
1	Transcranial direct current and repetitive magnetic stimulation may improve dysphagia in post-stroke patients [47]

Acupuncture

Acupuncture to treat post-stroke dysphagia is another somewhat controversial intervention method. Li et al. completed a meta-analysis including 29 RCTs evaluating the efficacy and safety of acupuncture for 2190 post-stroke patients. They noted that acupuncture resulted in significant short-term improvement of dysphagia compared to patients who did not receive rehabilitative therapy [48]. Additionally, high-intensity acupuncture (longer needle retention time and more treatment sessions) was noted to be more effective than low-intensity acupuncture.

Level of evidence	Conclusion
1	Acupuncture results in short-term dysphagia improvement in post-stroke patients [48]

Special Populations with Dysphagia

Head and Neck Cancer

Several studies have been conducted on measures that prevent or reduce the long-term side effects radiation and/or chemoradiation has on swallowing in head and neck cancer patients. These side effects include, but are not limited to: voice changes, mucositis, peripheral neuropathy, xerostomia, fibrosis, and trismus. Fibrosis impacts both the oral and pharyngeal muscles, contributing to reduced mobility and strength of musculature and structures during swallowing. While "late" effects are usually measured a year posttreatment, significant problems can develop years or decades after treatment has ended.

Educating chemoradiation patients on potential side effects and placing them on a targeted swallow exercise regime before, during, and after treatment results in improved quality of life over patients without a swallow rehabilitation prevention protocol [49]. Carnaby-Mann et al. found that patients who complied with a home-exercise swallowing program during and after chemoradiation had less risk of saliva reduction, trismus, and the need for enteral nutrition [50].

Level of evidence	Conclusion
2	Implementation of prophylactic swallowing exercises results in decreased post-radiation associated dysphagia and improved short- and long-term quality-of-life measures [50]

Cricopharyngeal Dysfunction

The surgical management of cricopharyngeal (CP) dysfunction includes botulinum toxin injections, dilation, and/or myotomy. CP myotomy can be performed either endoscopically or as an open procedure. Kocdor et al. performed a systematic review including 32 articles that compared these management strategies [51]. The "success rates" for improving dysphagia were highly variable but the means were 75% for botulinum toxin injection, 81% for dilation and 75% for myotomy. In logistic regression analysis, the success rate of myotomy was similar to dilation but significantly higher than botulinum toxin injection. They also found that endoscopic myotomy was 2.2 times as likely to be successful as open myotomy. Abu-Ghanem et al. completed a systematic review of 14 studies with 264 patients and found that the "success rates" for improving dysphagia were also highly variable (botulinum toxin 65%, dilation 42–100%, myotomy 27–90%). The dilation group was the only one to report a major complication of esophageal perforation and/or death [52]. Consistently, however, studies comparing treatment of CP dysfunction (not Zenker's diverticulum) report that heterogeneous outcome measurements preclude the ability to recommend specific clinical practices [52, 53].

Zenker's Diverticulum

Regarding methodology, a meta-analysis and systematic review by Parker and Misono compared the outcomes of endoscopic Zenker's diverticulectomy with carbon dioxide (CO_2) laser versus stapler. There were seven cohort study articles of 391 patients, but no randomized controlled trials in the review.

Outcomes favored stapler management with shorter nil per os (NPO) duration, length of stay, less fever, and less abnormal CXR. CO_2 management was associated with better swallowing outcomes and lower revision rate in this study but Verdonch and Morton found a higher failure rate in CO_2 laser myotomy (21.7%) versus stapler (18.9%) [54, 55]. Excluding dental injury, two separate analyses have shown that CO_2 laser-assisted diverticulectomy has a higher complication rate compared with endoscopic stapler management [54, 55].

When comparing open versus endoscopic approaches for Zenker's diverticulum, Verdonch and Morton found that open procedures had higher complications rates (11% open versus 7% endoscopic) but less failure (4.2% open versus 18.4% endoscopic). The most common complication for the open approach was recurrent laryngeal nerve injury (3.4%) and salivary fistula (3.7%) [55]. Albers et al. performed a review of 11 studies with 596 patients and found that endoscopic treatment had significantly reduced operating time, shorter length of hospitalization, faster PO intake, and lower complication rate than open treatment [56]. However, there was lower recurrence rate with the open approach.

Ishaq et al. performed a meta-analysis and systematic review evaluating the efficacy, safety, and limitations of flexible endoscopic treatment for Zenker's diverticulectomy. Twenty studies were included with 813 patients. There were no randomized controlled trials included. The rate of success overall was 91% (range 56.4–96.6%) but the requirement of multiple treatments was common. Adverse effects averaged 11.3% (8–16%). Perforation occurred in 41 patients (6.5%) and bleeding was common. Recurrence of symptoms or diverticulum averaged 10.5% (range 0–31.8%) [57]. Verdonch and Morton compared flexible versus rigid endoscopic management of Zenker's diverticulectomy. They found that flexible endoscopy had a higher failure rate (29%) and overall complication rate (14.3%) [55].

Level of evidence	Conclusion
3	Consistent clinical recommendations cannot be made on the treatment of CP dysfunction, as reported outcomes in the literature are varied. Endoscopic myotomy had fewer complications with a higher recurrence rate compared to open procedures [51–53]
3	Endoscopic procedures for Zenker's diverticulectomy showed reduced operating time, shorter hospitalization, and quicker PO intake clearance as compared to open Zenker's diverticulectomy [55, 56]
3	Compared to rigid diverticulectomy, flexible diverticulectomy exhibited higher failure and complication rates [55, 57]

Conclusion

In this chapter, we summarize the data that represents the best evidence in our current understanding of dysphagia evaluation and management. However, the body of literature for dysphagia care is ever evolving and high-quality studies in the future are needed to effectively guide best practices.

References

1. Bhattacharyya N. The prevalence of dysphagia among adults in the United States. Otolaryngol Head Neck Surg. 2014;151(5):765–9.
2. Cabré M, Serra-Prat M, Force L, Almirall J, Palomera E, Clave P. Oropharyngeal dysphagia is a risk factor for readmission for pneumonia in the very elderly persons: observational prospective study. J Gerontol Ser A Biol Med Sci. 2013;69A(3):330–7.
3. Roden DF, Altman KW. Causes of dysphagia among different age groups. Otolaryngol Clin N Am. 2013;46(6):965–87.

4. Crary M, Sura L, Madhavan A, Carnaby-Mann G. Dysphagia in the elderly: management and nutritional considerations. Clin Interv Aging. 2012;7:287–98.

5. Serra-Prat M, Hinojosa G, López D, Juan M, Fabré E, Voss DS, et al. Prevalence of oropharyngeal dysphagia and impaired safety and efficacy of swallow in independently living older persons. J Am Geriatr Soc. 2011;59(1):186–7.

6. Clavé P, Terré R, Kraa MD, Serra M. Approaching oropharyngeal dysphagia. Rev Esp Enferm Dig. 2004;96(2):119–31.

7. Luckmann R. Evidence-based medicine: how to practice and teach EBM, 2nd Edition: By David L. Sackett, Sharon E. Straus, W. Scott Richardson, William Rosenberg, and R. Brian Haynes, Churchill Livingstone, 2000. J Intensive Care Med. 2001;16(3):155–6.

8. Dysphagia. (2018, August 20). Retrieved from https://www.nidcd.nih.gov/health/dysphagia.

9. González-Fernández M, Humbert I, Winegrad H, Cappola AR, Fried LP. Dysphagia in old-old women: prevalence as determined according to self-report and the 3-ounce water swallowing test. J Am Geriatr Soc. 2014;62(4):716–20.

10. Newman R, Vilardell N, Clavé P, Speyer R. Erratum to: effect of bolus viscosity on the safety and efficacy of swallowing and the kinematics of the swallow response in patients with oropharyngeal dysphagia: White paper by the European Society for Swallowing Disorders (ESSD). Dysphagia. 2016;31(5):719.

11. Leonard RJ, White C, McKenzie S, Belafsky PC. Effects of bolus rheology on aspiration in patients with Dysphagia. J Acad Nutr Diet. 2014;114(4):590–4.

12. Kaneoka A, Pisegna JM, Saito H, Lo M, Felling K, Haga N, LaValley MP, Langmore SE. A systematic review and meta-analysis of pneumonia associated with thin liquid vs. thickened liquid intake in patients who aspirate. Clin Rehabil. 2016;31(8):1116–25.

13. Carlaw C, Finlayson H, Beggs K, et al. Outcomes of a pilot water protocol project in a rehabilitation setting. Dysphagia. 2012;27(3):297–306.

14. Murray J, Doeltgen S, Miller M, Scholten I. Does a water protocol improve the hydration and health status of individuals with thin liquid aspiration following stroke? A randomized controlled trial. Dysphagia. 2016;31(3):424–33.

15. Becker DL, Tews LK, Lemke JH. An oral water protocol in rehabilitation patients with dysphagia for liquids. 2008, ASHA convention handouts.

16. Kenedi H, Campbell V, Reynolds J. Implementing oral care & free water protocol studies in acute care: a collaborative model. 2013, ASHA convention handouts.

17. Michou E, Mastan A, Ahmed S, Mistry S, Hamdy S. Examining the role of carbonation and temperature on water swallowing performance: a swallowing reaction-time study. Chem Senses. 2012;37(9):799–807.

18. Rofes L, Arreola V, Martin A, Clavé P. Effect of oral piperine on the swallow response of patients with oropharyngeal dysphagia. J Gastroenterol. 2014;49(12):1517–23.

19. Huggins PS, Tuomi SK, Young C. Effects of nasogastric tubes on the young, normal swallowing mechanism. Dysphagia. 1999;14(3):157–61.

20. Pryor LN, Ward EC, Cornwell PL, O'Connor SN, Finnis ME, Chapman MJ. Impact of nasogastric tubes on swallowing physiology in older, healthy subjects: a randomized controlled crossover trial. Clin Nutr. 2015;34(4):572–8.

21. O'Dea MB, Langmore SE, Krisciunas GP, Walsh M, Zanchetti LL, Scheel R, et al. Effect of lidocaine on swallowing during FEES in patients with dysphagia. Ann Otol Rhinol Laryngol. 2015;124(7):537–44.

22. Kamarunas EE, Mccullough GH, Guidry TJ, Mennemeier M, Schluterman K. Effects of topical nasal anesthetic on fiberoptic endoscopic examination of swallowing with sensory testing (FEESST). Dysphagia. 2013;29(1):33–43.

23. Fife TA, Butler SG, Langmore SE, Lester S, Wright SC, Kemp S, Grace-Martin K, Lintzenich CR. Use of topical nasal anesthesia during flexible endoscopic evaluation of swallowing in dysphagic patients. Ann Otol Rhinol Laryngol. 2015;124(3):206–11.

24. Hernandez EG, Gozdzikowska K, Apperley O, Huckabee M. Effect of topical nasal anesthetic on swallowing in healthy adults: a double-blind, high-resolution manometry study. Laryngoscope. 2017;128(6):1335–9.

25. Kertscher B, Speyer R, Palmieri M, Plant C. Bedside screening to detect oropharyngeal dysphagia in patients with neurological disorders: an updated systematic review. Dysphagia. 2014;29:204–12.

26. Warnecke T, Im S, Kaiser C, Hamacher C, Oelenberg S, Dziewas R. Aspiration and dysphagia screening in acute stroke—The Gugging Swallowing Screen revisited. Eur J Neurol. 2017;24(4):594–601.

27. Robbins J, Coyle J, Rosenbek J, Roecker E, Wood J. Differentiation of normal and abnormal airway protection during swallowing using the Penetration-Aspiration Scale. Dysphagia. 1999;14:228–32.

28. Steele CM, Grace-Martin K. Reflections of clinical and statistical use of the Penetration-Aspiration scale. Dysphagia. 2017;32:601–16.

29. Baijens L, Barikroo A, Pilz W. Intrarater and interrater reliability for measurements in videofluoroscopy of swallowing. Eur J Radiol. 2013;82:1683–95.

30. Butler SG, Markley L, Sanders B, Stuart A. Reliability of the Penetration-Aspiration scale with flexible endoscopic evaluation of swallowing. Ann Otol Rhinol Laryngol. 2015;124(6):480–3.

31. Scharitzer M, Roesner I, Pokieser P, Weber M, Denk-Linnert DM. Simultaneous radiological and fiberendoscopic evaluation of swallowing ("SIRFES") in patients after surgery of oropharyngeal/laryngeal cancer and postoperative dysphagia. Dysphagia. 2019;34:852–61.

32. Rommel N, Hamdy S. Oropharyngeal dysphagia: manifestations and diagnosis. Nat Rev Gastroenterol Hepatol. 2016;13:49–59.

33. Bath PM, Lee HS, Everton LF. Swallowing therapy for dysphagia in acute and subacute stroke. Stroke. 2019;50(3):e46–e47.

34. Park J, An D, Oh D, Chang M. Effect of chin tuck against resistance exercise on patients with dysphagia following stroke: a randomized pilot study. NeuroRehabilitation. 2018;42(2):191–7.
35. Chen Z, Wei X, Li F, He P, Huang X, Zhang F, et al. Tracheal traction exercise reduces the occurrence of postoperative dysphagia after anterior cervical spine surgery. Spine. 2012;37(15):1292–6.
36. Moon J, Hahm S, Won YS, Cho H. The effects of tongue pressure strength and accuracy training on tongue pressure strength, swallowing function, and quality of life in subacute stroke patients with dysphagia. Int J Rehabil Res. 2018;41(3):204–10.
37. Fujimaki Y, Tsunoda K, Kobayashi R, et al. Independent exercise for glottal incompetence to improve vocal problems and prevent aspiration pneumonia in the elderly: a randomized controlled trial. Clin Rehabil. 31(8):1049–56.
38. Terré R, Mearin F. Effectiveness of chin-down posture to prevent tracheal aspiration in dysphagia secondary to acquired brain injury. A videofluoroscopy study. Neurogastroenterol Motil. 2012;24(5):414–9. e206
39. Carnaby-Mann GD, Crary MA. Examining the evidence on neuromuscular electrical stimulation for swallowing. Arch Otolaryngol Head Neck Surg. 2007;133(6):564–71.
40. Park JW, Oh JC, Lee HJ, Park SJ, Yoon TS, Kwon BS. Effortful swallowing training coupled with electrical stimulation leads to an increase in hyoid elevation during swallowing. Dysphagia. 2009;24(3):296–301.
41. Chen Y-W, Chang K-H, Chen H-C, Liang W-M, Wang Y-H, Lin Y-N. The effects of surface neuromuscular electrical stimulation on post-stoke dysphagia: a systematic review and meta-analysis. Clin Rehabil. 2016;30(1):24–35.
42. Tan C, Liu Y, Li W, Liu J, Chen L. Transcutaneous neuromuscular electrical stimulation can improve swallowing function in patients with dysphagia caused by non-stroke diseases: a meta-analysis. J Oral Rehabil. 2013;40(6):472–80.
43. Clark H, Lazarus C, Arvedson J, Schooling T, Frymark T. Evidence-based systematic review: effects of neuromuscular electrical stimulation on swallowing and neural activation. Am J Speech Lang Pathol. 2009;18:361–75.
44. Ortega O, Rofes L, Martin A, Arreola V, López I, Clavé P. A comparative study between two sensory stimulation strategies after two weeks treatment on older patients with oropharyngeal dysphagia. Dysphagia. 2016;31(5):706–16.
45. Konecny P, Elfmark M. Electrical stimulation of hyoid muscles in post-stroke dysphagia. Biomed Pap Med Fac Univ Palacky Olomouc Czech Repub. 2018;162(1):40–2.
46. Lim K, Lee H, Lim S, Choi Y. Neuromuscular electrical and thermal-tactile stimulation for dysphagia caused by stroke: a randomized controlled trial. J Rehabil Med. 2009;41(3):174–8.

47. Pisegna JM, Kaneoka A, Pearson WG Jr, Kumar S, Langmore SE. Effects of non-invasive brain stimulation on post-stroke dysphagia: a systematic review and meta-analysis of randomized controlled trials. Clin Neurophysiol. 2016;127:956–68.

48. Li L, Deng K, Qu Y. Acupuncture treatment for post-stroke dysphagia: an update meta-analysis of randomized controlled trials. Chin J Integr Med. 2018;24(9):686–95.

49. Kraaijenga SA, Molen LV, Jacobi I, Hamming-Vrieze O, Hilgers FJ, Van Den Brekel MWM. Prospective clinical study on long-term swallowing function and voice quality in advanced head and neck cancer patients treated with concurrent chemoradiotherapy and preventive swallowing exercises. Eur Arch Otorhinolaryngol. 2014;272(11):3521–31.

50. Carnaby-Mann G, Crary MA, Schmalfuss I, Amdur R. "Pharyngocise": randomized controlled trial of preventative exercises to maintain muscle structure and swallowing function during head-and-neck chemoradiotherapy. Int J Radiat Oncol Biol Phys. 2012;83(1):210–9.

51. Kocdor P, Siegel ER, Tulunay-Ugur OE. Cricopharyngeal dysfunction: a systematic review comparing outcomes of dilatation, botulinum toxin injection, and myotomy. Laryngoscope. 2016;126(1):135–41.

52. Abu-Ghanem S, Sung C, Junlapan A, Kearney A, Direnzo E, Dewan K, Damrose EJ. Endoscopic management of postradiation dysphagia in head and neck cancer patients: a systematic review. Ann Otol Rhinol Laryngol. 2019;128(8):767–73.

53. Knigge MA, Thibeault SL. Swallowing outcomes after cricopharyngeal myotomy: a systematic review. Head Neck. 2018;40(1):203–12.

54. Parker NP, Misono S. Carbon dioxide laser versus stapler-assisted endoscopic Zenker's diverticulotomy: a systematic review and meta-analysis. Otolaryngol Head Neck Surg. 2014;150(5):750–3.

55. Verdonck J, Morton RP. Systematic review on treatment of Zenker's diverticulum. Eur Arch Otorhinolaryngol. 2015;272(11):3095–107.

56. Albers DV, Kondo A, Bernardo WM, Sakai P, et al. Endoscopic versus surgical approach in the treatment of Zenker's diverticulum: systematic review and meta-analysis. Endosc Int Open. 2016;4(6):E678–86.

57. Ishaq S, Hassan C, Antonello A, et al. Flexible endoscopic treatment for Zenker's diverticulum: a systematic review and meta-analysis. Gastrointest Endosc. 2016;83(6):1076–89.

Index

© Springer Nature Switzerland AG 2021
D. E. Rosow, C. M. Ivey (eds.), *Evidence-Based Laryngology*,
https://doi.org/10.1007/978-3-030-58494-8